One Minute MIGRAINE Diary

Eyes Off! This Information Is Private.

This Journal Belongs To

If Found, Please Return To

AF808769

WWW.ONEMINUTEMIGRAINEDIARY.COM

One Minute MIGRAINE Diary

Training and information on how to use this diary can be found at:

WWW.ONEMINUTEMIGRAINEDIARY.COM

Book Media Services

One Minute MIGRAINE Diary

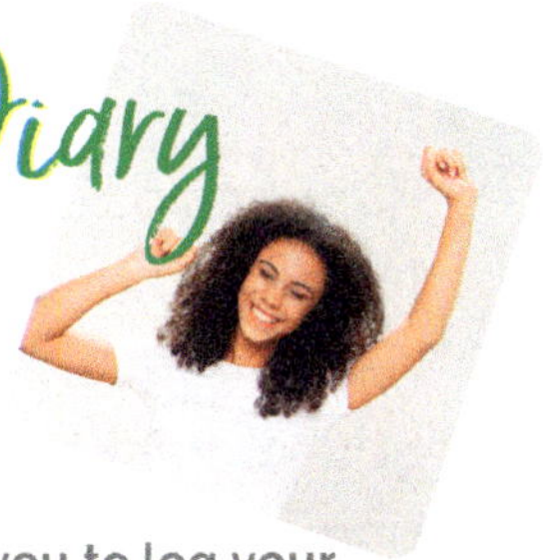

Congratulations on taking the time to track your headaches.Tracking leads to Treating!

I hope the One Minute Migraine Diary makes it easy for you to log your headaches and other migraine symptoms, medication use, and a wide range of triggers (moods, weather, diet, etc.) that may affect the occurrence of headaches/migraines.

This diary is customizable to suit the things you'd like to track.
Important Features Include:

- ✓ Personal Analytical Report to help you confirm and manage lifestyle factors associated with your migraine attacks
- ✓ Identify potential triggers, protectors, and warning signs
- ✓ Extensive diary of your attack symptoms
- ✓ Medications Log
- ✓ Track the effect of migraine on your activities, which may be useful for discussions with your doctor, employer, etc.

Are you ready to:

Say goodbye to unpredictability...
Start taking control of your headaches and find some predictability within your headache journey...
Create your headache breakthrough plan
Break free from headaches and unleash your full potential!
Create the life you know you were meant to live, exactly on your own terms

For Ultimate "Headache Tracking and Healing Breakthrough" Sign up for Migraine Factor X Challenge NOW: www.migrainefactorx.com/education

facebook.com/MigraineFactorx
facebook.com/groups/migrainediary

WWW.ONEMINUTEMIGRAINEDIARY.COM

HOW IT ALL BEGAN

Kam has occasional migraines but this gene has magnified in her daughter who experiences more intense and frequent headaches than her mom. Luckily, Kam's husband is a neurologist hence their daughter has access to professional, personalized care and support.

Kam founded migrainefactorx.com a website dedicated to providing resources to help migraine warriors around the world who do not have access to on-demand medical advice which her daughter was privileged to have as her father helped her navigate migraines on a day to day basis.

Migraine FactorX's mission is to:
1 Help reduce the frequency and intensity of migraine through education and support. Research proves that migraine education helps reduces migraines [Source: US National Library of Medicine]. Check out our migraine education program at migrainefactorx.com/education

2 To provide resources for proper tracking and treatment of headaches. (One Minute Migraine Diary)

3 To provide information about the latest research opportunities and to help connect migraine warriors with appropriate research studies. Check out research studies that are currently enrolling at migrainefactorx.com/research

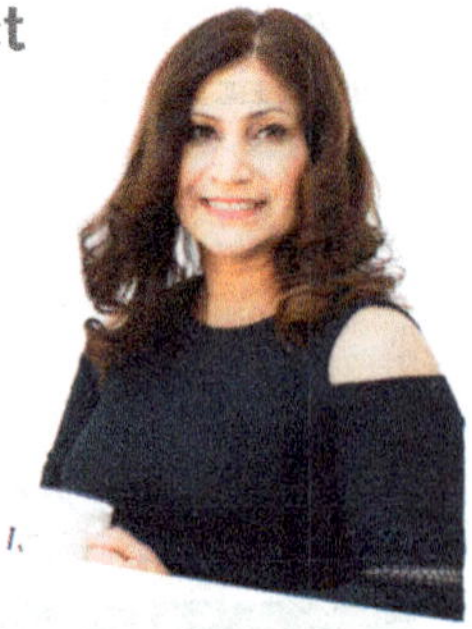

WWW.ONEMINUTEMIGRAINEDIARY.COM

DEDICATION

We would like to thank Dr. Rajiv Aggarwal as without his guidance this resource would not have been possible.

We are honored to have Dr. Aggrwal's support on an ongoing basis. His feedback and insights were valuable and ensured that we had appropriate triggers and factors available in the diary, making sure that the most important information for decision making is recorded and also to ensure that none of the hidden triggers were missed.

Rajiv Kumar Aggarwal, MD is a neurologist with Minneapolis Clinic of Neurology. His primary location is in Burnsville, MN. He has more than 20 years of experience in Migraine Disorders, Sleep Medicine, and General Neurology.

He serves on the advisory board of Migraine FactorX the parent organization behind the one minute migraine diary.

Dr. Rajiv Aggarwal is the principal investigator for multiple migraine research studies and brings the latest in headache education and research to our community.

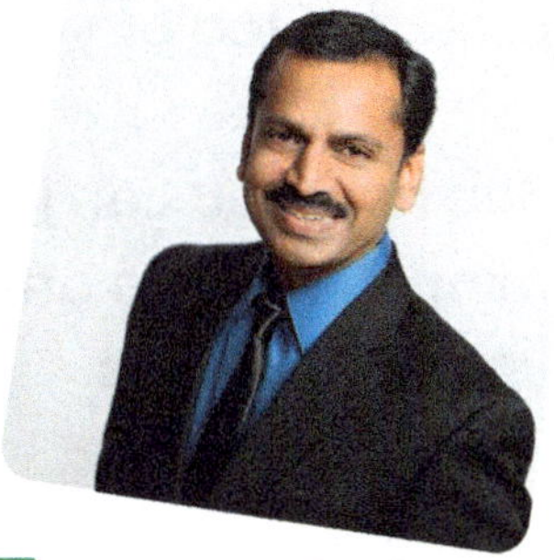

INTRODUCTION

Hey there!

We are so excited that you've decided to pick up this valuable resource.

A daily headache diary is one of the most important tools for understanding and treating headaches.

A well-documented headache diary helps to:

- ✓ Monitor the frequency, duration, and severity of headaches over time
- ✓ Identify patterns that may help determine triggers and improve treatment
- ✓ Track medication use and response
- ✓ Review diary to understand what has worked and what has not

A headache trigger tracker/ diary can help plan treatment and manage your headaches.

Our mission is to take the headache out of maintaining an effective log of your headaches.

See how you can just spend a minute a day to effectively log your headaches.

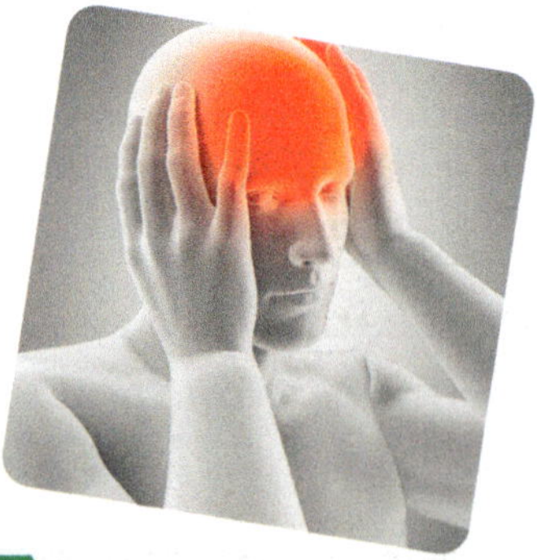

MY HEADACHE *Diary*

Thank you for choosing the One Minute Migraine diary to document your headaches. **Commit to using this diary every day for atleast 90 days which is 3 months.** Record every headache, including mild headaches.

This diary is designed to track important details such as:

✓ **Date & Time** when the headache and any other symptoms began and ended. Women should keep track of their menstrual cycle and note if any headaches occurred before or during menstruation.

✓ **Severity**: Rate your pain on a scale from 1-10, with 1 being mild and 10 being the most severe pain. Pain between 4-7 is considered moderate.

✓ **Triggers**: Take note of all food & beverage consumed in the last 24 hours. Any of the potential items on the trigger list consumed within a 24-hour period prior to the onset of headache could be a trigger.

✓ **Associated Symptoms**: Any other symptoms that occurred before, during, or after the headache, including nausea, vomiting, light and noise sensitivity, worsening of the headache when physically active, lightheadedness, or dizziness. Note if there were any changes in your vision, sensation, speech, etc., and how long this lasted.

✓ **Treatment**: Record if any medication was taken and the dose. Was the medication taken within one hour of headache onset or later into the episode? Did the headache improve or resolve with treatment?

✓ **Duration**: Estimate how long the headache lasted, even if you did not take any medication.

✓ **Remedies and Relief:** Note any therapeutic, OTC, RX, supplements, or preventative medications that provide relief.

WWW.ONEMINUTEMIGRAINEDIARY.COM

BENEFITS OF Diary

You will begin to see a pattern after several months of documenting your headache diary. This will allow you to identify your triggers. Avoiding the triggers can help reduce the frequency of migraine attacks.

Things to pay attention to:

- ✓ **Combination of triggers** Often, it is the combination of triggers that can lead to a migraine. For example, the combination of lack of sleep, eating chocolates, and a change in the barometric pressure can lead to an attack. Therefore, there may be times when you have exposure to a certain food trigger, such as nuts, but not experience a headache every time after consuming this food, but it can still be a trigger.

- ✓ **Food Triggers**: You may notice a pattern of certain food or beverages that were consumed within the 24-hour period before a migraine. These items are considered potential triggers. Try to eliminate these items from your diet for a month and continue to track your symptoms.

- ✓ **Lifestyle Triggers:** Notice your sleep, stress levels, water consumption exercise habits, and changes in your routine when tracking your headaches and reviewing your diary.

- ✓ **Hormonal Triggers:** For women, notice if there is a pattern of headaches before or during your menstrual cycle. Migraines which are related to menstruation most commonly occur 2 days before and up to 2 days into the cycle.

WWW.ONEMINUTEMIGRAINEDIARY.COM

PERSONAL Notes

This page is intentionally left blank for you to take notes about your intentions of using this diary and how do you plan to use it.

✓ I commit to making my health better by working towards understanding my migraines better. Keeping a daily log of headaches is the first step towards headache management .

WWW.ONEMINUTEMIGRAINEDIARY.COM

PERSONAL *Notes*

Take notes about your intentions of using this diary and how do you plan to use it.

✓ I commit to making my health better by working towards understanding my migraines better. Keeping a daily log of headaches is the first step towards headache management .

WWW.ONEMINUTEMIGRAINEDIARY.COM

TRIGGER LIST *Key*

It is important to note that most of the information about possible food triggers of headache come from patient self-reporting and not from randomized scientific studies. The most common foods and drinks reported to be potential headache triggers are included below.

✓ **While recording in the headache diary, feel free to just use the KEY for ease of use**

Key	Description	Suggested Replacement
Alcohol	Alcoholic Beverages - Red Wine, Beer, Whiskey, Scotch, Champagne, Cocktails etc	Non alcoholic drinks
Artificial Sweetener	Artificial Sweeteners (i.e. aspartame)	Stevia, regular sugar
Beans	Fava, Lima, Kidney , Garbenzo, Italian, Pole, Broad, Navy, Pinto, Snow Peas, and Dried Beans and Peas	Lentils
Caffine	Caffeinated Beverages	Decaffeinated drinks
Cheese	Breads/crackers containing cheese	Crackers/breads without cheese
Cheese	Cheese: Ripened or Aged Cheeses (i.e. Emmentaler,Brie, Camembert Blue Cheese, Cheddar, English Stilton, Feta, Gorgonzola, Mozzarella, Muenster, Parmesan, Swiss)	Fresh cheeses including feta, ricotta, goat cheese
Cheese	Pizza	Market fresh wraps
Chocolate	Chocolate	Caramel
Condiments	Seasoned Salt	Regular salt
Condiments	Sour Cream	Fresh cream
Condiments	Soy Sauce	Avoid
Fermented Foods	Fermented, pickled (pickles, olives, sauerkraut) or marinated foods	Avoid
Fruits	Bananas, Oranges, Figs, Raisins, Papayas,Avocados, Red Plums	Berries, grapes, apples
Fruits	Citrus Fruits - (orange, grapefruit, tangerine etc) Bananas, Papaya, Red Plums, Kiwi, and Pineapple	Berries, grapes, apples
MSG	MSG	Salt and pepper
Nuts	Nuts -any kind: Peanuts cashews, almonds, walnuts, pistachio etc Peanut Butter	Sunflower seeds, Sunflower seed butter
Other	Herring	Other kind of fish
Other	Meat Tenderizers	Salt and pepper
Processed Meat	Chicken Liver	Unprocessed meat, fish
Processed Meats	Processed Meats contain nitrate/nitrite: Sausage, bologna, pepperoni, salami, hot dogs	Avoid
Yeast	Sourdough Bread fresh baked yeast goods (donuts, cakes, homemade breads, and rolls)	Regular bread

*** Please note this is not a complete list of all triggers. Understanding and discovering your triggers require you to pay close attention to food intake and symptoms experienced within a span of 24 hours.

PERSONAL *triggers*

Take notes about your frequent triggers and possible replacements or management

✓ **I commit to making my health a priority and will try to find a replacement for my triggers.**

PERSONAL *triggers*

Take notes about your frequent triggers and possible replacements or management

✓ I commit to making my health a priority and will try to find a replacement for my triggers.

PERSONAL *triggers*

Take notes about your frequent triggers and possible replacements or management

✓ **I commit to making my health a priority and will try to find a replacement for my triggers.**

WWW.ONEMINUTEMIGRAINEDIARY.COM

HOW TO USE THIS Diary

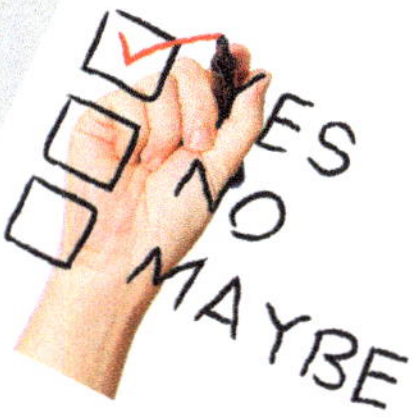

- Take a minute every day to record your headaches.
- Each week, take a few minutes to update the monthly and annual reports found at the very end of the diary.
- Each month take time to review monthly and annual trends.
- The recording is quite simple where you just have to circle the option that best represents your state.
- Follow the food trigger key list to record appropriately. You can add additional items to the food key list if needed.
- Use the notes section and the empty space within each section to record additional data, if required.
- Record on the same day, do not wait to record the data about your headaches. It is very important to accurately record the duration, time, severity, type, triggers, symptoms, and pain relievers accurately.

Good Deal? Let's get started.

Are you ready to roll?

WWW.ONEMINUTEMIGRAINEDIARY.COM

EXAMPLE Sheets

The following pages provide you with examples of how to fill in the daily, annual, and monthly sheets to accurately record your migraines. **Monthly and annual sheets are located at the very end of this diary in order to help you locate them easily.**

Daily Sheet is Divided into THREE SECTIONS: General Information section, Triggers and Symptoms section and Remedies and Relief section

✓ **GENERAL SECTION:** This section includes general information about your headaches such as - Date, day, start time, end time, duration, pain scale, pain location, pain type, monthly periods (women), birth control pills (women), weather (remember to record barometric pressure and temperature), exposure to excessive lights, sounds and smell, stress, missed meals and water intake. **Put a check or circle all that apply. Try not to ignore answering the question within this section. The idea is to for a second if the given choice is applicable to your migraine/headache.**

✓ **TRIGGER AND SYMPTOMS SECTION:** This section includes information specific to triggers and symptoms related to migraines. This section is further divided into five sub-sections - Foods Consumed, Prodrome Symptoms, Symptoms, Aura, and Notes. **The most common choices are included in each sub-section, and space is provided to add your own.** **Foods Consumed** - In this section record all foods consumed within the last 24 hours from the onset of the headache. Refer to the key for a detailed list of foods, **Prodrome Section**- Record any symptoms that occur 1-2 hours before the actual headache. **Aura Section**- Record any symptoms that occur 20-30 mins before the actual headache. If you do not experience prodrome or aura you can ignore this section, however, we do recommend you to reflect on this section for a second or two, **Symptoms and Notes Section** is provided to complete your headache log.

✓ **REMEDIES AND RELIEF SECTION:** In this section record any Natural, Over-the-Counter (OTC), or prescription (Rx) remedies you tried during an acute migraine attack. **Record if you took the Rx medication within 1 hour of pain onset and if it helped to relieve the pain.** Any ongoing preventive medications and supplements you take are also recorded in this section.

*** **Please remember to record the impact your migraine had on your daily activities.**

WWW.ONEMINUTEMIGRAINEDIARY.COM

One Minute MIGRAINE Diary

Date : *Jan 02, 2022*

Start Time : *8:00 AM* End Time : *11:00 AM* Duration : *3 HRS*

PAIN SCALE [1-10]: 1 2 3 4 5 6 7 8 9 10 — MILD, MODERATE, SEVERE (8 circled)

MENSTRUAL PERIOD: YES NO (NO marked)

Birth Control Pills: YES NO (NO marked)

PAIN TYPE: Stabbing, Burning, Pulsating, Shocking, Pressure, Pounding (Pounding circled)

WATER

SLEEP

MISSED MEALS: YES NO (NO marked)

PAIN LOCATION: FRONT, BACK, LEFT, RIGHT, TOP (RIGHT and TOP marked)

WEATHER: *30.22* *15* ° TEMP

STRESS: YES NO (NO marked)

LIGHTS: YES NO (NO marked)

SOUNDS: YES NO (NO marked)

SMELLS: YES NO (NO marked)

FOODS CONSUMED (within last 24 hours)

- [x] Alcohol
- [ ] Artificial Sweetener
- [ ] Beans
- [ ] Caffeine
- [ ] Cheese
- [x] Chocolate
- [ ] Fermented Foods
- [ ] MSG
- [ ] Non Friendly Fruits
- [x] Nuts
- [ ] Processed Meats

PRODROME (1-2 hours before headache)

- [ ] Excessive Thirst
- [ ] Excessive Yawning
- [x] Face Sensitivity
- [ ] Irritability
- [ ] Light Sensitivity
- [x] Neck Tightness
- [ ] Unexplained Fatigue
- [ ] Visual Disturbances

SYMPTOMS

- [ ] Distorted Vision
- [x] Dizziness
- [ ] Irritability
- [x] Light-headedness
- [ ] Light Sensitivity
- [ ] Malaise
- [ ] Nasal Congestion
- [x] Nausea/Vomiting
- [ ] Sound Sensitivity
- [ ] Tender Scalp

AURA (20-30 mins before)

- [ ] Black Spots
- [ ] Flashing Lights
- [ ] Lack of Vision
- [x] Numbness FACE ARM LEG (FACE circled)
- [ ] Zig Zag Lines
- [ ] *Jagged arc of light to the left*

TRIGGER & SYMPTOM NOTES

Party food is a NO-NO

REMEDIES

(NATURAL)

- [ ] Acupuncture
- [ ] Acupressure
- [ ] Caffeine
- [ ] Dark Room
- [x] Hot Compress
- [ ] Hydration
- [ ] Ice Pack
- [ ] Massage
- [x] Relaxation
- [x] Silence
- [ ] Walk

(OTC- COUNTER MEDS)

- [ ] Excedrin
- [ ] Ibuprofen
- [ ] Tylenol

(Rx - PREVENTIVE)

- [ ] Amitriptyline
- [ ] Atenolol
- [x] Gabapentin
- [ ] Nurtriptyline
- [ ] Propranolol
- [ ] Topamax
- [ ] Valproate

(Rx - RELIEF)

- [ ] Naproxin
- [x] Nurtec
- [ ] Sumatriptan
- [ ] Rizatriptan
- [ ] Ubrelvy

(SUPPLEMENTS)

- [x] B2
- [ ] Butterbur
- [ ] Feverfew
- [x] Magnesium

WITHIN 1 HR OF PAIN: YES NO (YES circled)

PAIN RELIEF: YES NO (NO circled)

REMEDY NOTES

Nurtec did its MAGIC in 2 hrs!

IMPACT ON DAILY ACTIVITIES: NONE | MILD | MODERATE | SEVERE (MODERATE circled)

WWW.ONEMINUTEMIGRAINEDIARY.COM

EXAMPLE *Sheets*

Each week, take a few minutes to update the monthly and annual reports. If you can, try to record them on the day you experience headaches. **Monthly and annual sheets are located at the very end of this diary in order to help you locate them easily.**

The Monthly Tracking Sheet is Divided into FIVE MAIN SECTIONS: Month, Day, Severity of Headaches, Daily Top Triggers, Monthly Top Triggers, and Monthly Totals.

- ✓ **MONTH SECTION:** Fill in the month that you will be tracking. **Dates from 1-31 are already filled in for you.**
- ✓ **KEY SECTION:** Fill in the key for the day and date when you had a headache. Remember mild (M) is 1-3, moderate (MO) is 4-7, and severe (S) is 8-10.
- ✓ **TOP TRIGGER SECTION:** This section is included to summarize the top triggers that you identified were responsible for this headache.
- ✓ **MONTHLY TOP TRIGGER SECTION:** This section is included to summarize the top triggers that seem to repeat throughout the month.
- ✓ **MONTHLY TOTALS:** Count the number of entries in the KEY section to get a total for the number of migraines you had in that month.

The Annual Tracking Sheet is Divided into FIVE MAIN SECTIONS: Year, Month, Days, Severity of Headaches, Monthly and Annual Top Triggers, Monthly, and Annual Totals.

- ✓ **ANNUAL SECTION:** Fill in the Year that you will be tracking. **Dates from 1-31 and months from Jan-Dec are already filled in for you. In order to record your migraine, just record the severity in the correct column.** Start with the column that represents the current month and scroll down to the correct row that represents the current day and record.
- ✓ **TOP MONTHLY AND ANNUAL TRIGGERS SECTION:** This section is to the left of the day (1-31) and uses numbers (1-12) which represent months and not days. Record top triggers for the month here. The top annual triggers section is right below, just pen your very top triggers here.
- ✓ **MONTHLY AND ANNUAL TOTALS SECTION:** The count for each month and an annual count section is available to get a monthly and annual total for your migraine.

*** **Monthly and Annual Sheets provide the complete snapshot of your migraines.**

WWW.ONEMINUTEMIGRAINEDIARY.COM

MONTHLY MIGRAINE Report

Month/ Year : Jan 2022

KEY : M (Mild) MO(Moderate) S(Severe)

MONTH		KEY	TOP DAILY TRIGGERS
	1		
TOP MONTHLY TRIGGERS	2		
	3		
	4	S	Nuts, Chocolate, Alcohol
	5		
	6		
Alcohol, Sleep & Nuts	7	MO	Menstrual. Period, Sleep
	8		
	9		
	10		
	11		
	12		
	13	S	Barometric, Sleep
	14		
	15		
	16		
	17	MO	Nuts, Chocolate, Alcohol
	18		
	19		
	20		
	21	MO	Nuts, Chocolate, Alcohol
	22		
	23		
	24	MO	Barometric , Nuts, Alcohol
	25		
	26	MO	Barometric , Sleep, Alcohol
	27	S	MSG , Stress, Sleep
	28		
	29	S	Stress , Fruits, Sleep
	30		
	31		

MONTHLY TOTAL: 9

ANNUAL MIGRAINE *Report*

Year : 2021

KEY : M (Mild) MO(Moderate) S(Severe)

TOP MONTHLY TRIGGERS		J	F	M	A	M	J	J	A	S	O	N	D
Nuts, Chocolate, Alcohol	1	S											
Nuts, Chocolate, Alcohol	2										MO		
Barometric, Sleep	3												
Menstrual. Period, Sleep	4												S
Barometric , Sleep, Alcohol	5	S					S						
MSG , Stress, Sleep	6			MO					MO		S		
	7										MO		MO
Stress , Fruits, Sleep	8	MO							MO				
	9						MO						
Barometric , Nuts, Alcohol	10				MO								
Nuts, Chocolate, Alcohol	11												
Nuts, Chocolate, Alcohol	12				MO								S
TOP ANNUAL TRIGGERS	13	S											
	14				S								
	15		S		S		S						
	16		S										MO
Alcohol, Nuts, Sleep	17												
	18						MO						
	19		MO										
	20												MO
	21	MO										MO	
	22			S									
	23												MO
	24												
	25		S									S	MO
	26					MO							S
	27	S										S	S
	28		MO			MO							
	29												
	30											MO	
	31												
TOTAL / MONTH		6	5	2	4	2	4		2		3	4	9

GRAND TOTAL: 36

WWW.ONEMINUTEMIGRAINEDIARY.COM

One Minute MIGRAINE Diary

Fill Up Your Gratitude Jar!

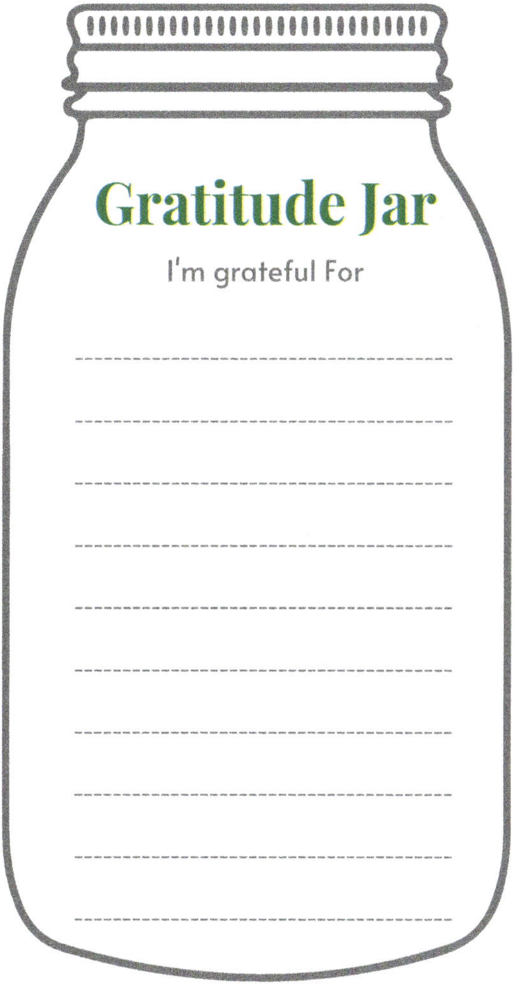

Gratitude lights up the same part of the brain that is associated with the pain relief experienced by viewing a loved one

One Minute MIGRAINE Diary

Fill Up Your Gratitude Jar!

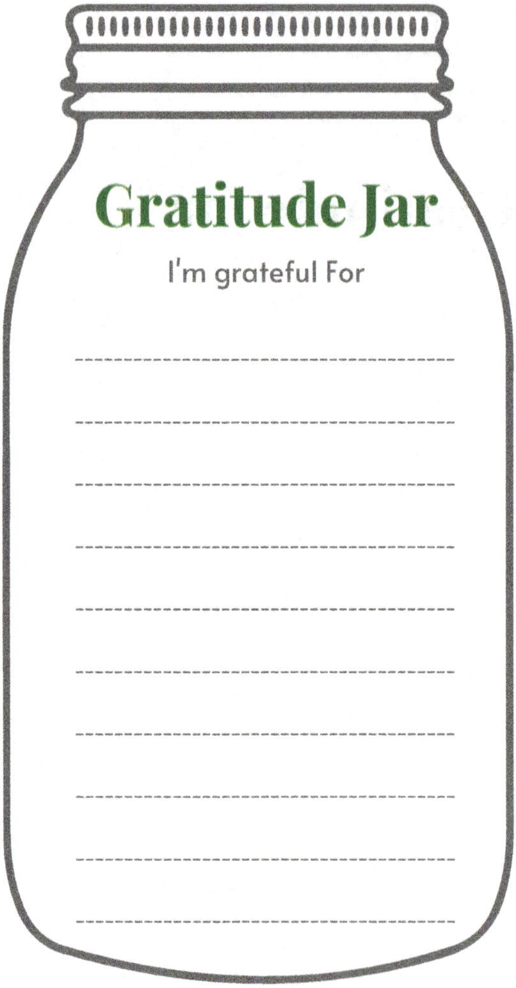

Gratitude lights up the same part of the brain that is associated with the pain relief experienced by viewing a loved one

One Minute MIGRAINE Diary

Month

Migraine Tracking Prompts, Reflections and Assessments To Help You Track and Manage Your Migraines

WWW.ONEMINUTEMIGRAINEDIARY.COM

I am not my pain
My pain does not define me
I am not my pain
I am not defined by my pain
I am not my pain
I am strong, capable and confident

Book MEDIA Services

One Minute MIGRAINE Diary

Date : ______________________

Start Time : ______________ End Time : ____________ Duration : ______

PAIN SCALE [1-10]	MENSTRUAL PERIOD	PAIN TYPE	WATER
1 2 3 4 5 6 7 8 9 10 MILD MODERATE SEVERE	YES NO Birth Control Pills YES NO	Stabbing Burning Pulsating Shocking Pressure Pounding **SLEEP**	**MISSED MEALS** YES NO
PAIN LOCATION FRONT BACK LEFT RIGHT TOP		**WEATHER** TEMP °	**STRESS** YES NO
		LIGHTS YES NO **SOUNDS** YES NO	**SMELLS** YES NO

FOODS CONSUMED (within last 24 hours)	PRODROME (1-2 hours before headache)	SYMPTOMS	AURA (20-30 mins before)
☐ Alcohol	☐ Excessive Thirst	☐ Distorted Vision	☐ Black Spots
☐ Artificial Sweetener	☐ Excessive Yawning	☐ Dizziness	☐ Flashing Lights
☐ Beans	☐ Face Sensitivity	☐ Irritability	☐ Lack of Vision
☐ Caffeine	☐ Irritability	☐ Light-headedness	☐ Numbness FACE ARM LEG
☐ Cheese	☐ Light Sensitivity	☐ Light Sensitivity	☐ Zig Zag Lines
☐ Chocolate	☐ Neck Tightness	☐ Malaise	☐
☐ Fermented Foods	☐ Unexplained Fatigue	☐ Nasal Congestion	☐
☐ MSG	☐ Visual Disturbances	☐ Nausea/Vomiting	**TRIGGER & SYMPTOM NOTES**
☐ Non Friendly Fruits	☐	☐ Sound Sensitivity	
☐ Nuts	☐	☐ Tender Scalp	
☐ Processed Meats	☐	☐	
☐	☐	☐	
☐	☐	☐	
☐	☐		

REMEDIES

(NATURAL)		(OTC- COUNTER MEDS)	(Rx - PREVENTIVE)	(Rx - RELIEF)	(SUPPLEMENTS)
☐ Acupuncture	☐ Ice Pack	☐ Excedrin	☐ Amitriptyline	☐ Naproxin	☐ B2
☐ Acupressure	☐ Massage	☐ Ibuprofen	☐ Atenolol	☐ Nurtec	☐ Butterbur
☐ Caffeine	☐ Relaxation	☐ Tylenol	☐ Gabapentin	☐ Sumatriptan	☐ Feverfew
☐ Dark Room	☐ Silence	☐	☐ Nurtriptyline	☐ Rizatriptan	☐ Magnesium
☐ Hot Compress	☐ Walk	☐	☐ Propranolol	☐ Ubrelvy	☐
☐ Hydration	☐	☐	☐ Topamax	☐	☐
☐	☐	☐	☐ Valproate	☐	☐
☐	☐	☐	☐	WITHIN 1 HR OF PAIN YES NO	PAIN RELIEF YES NO
☐	☐	☐	☐		

REMEDY NOTES

IMPACT ON DAILY ACTIVITIES

NONE | MILD | MODERATE | SEVERE

WWW.ONEMINUTEMIGRAINEDIARY.COM

One Minute MIGRAINE Diary

Date : ______________________

Start Time : ________________ End Time : ______________ Duration : ________

PAIN SCALE [1-10]	MENSTRUAL PERIOD	PAIN TYPE	WATER
1 2 3 4 5 6 7 8 9 10 MILD MODERATE SEVERE	YES NO Birth Control Pills YES NO	Stabbing Burning Pulsating Shocking Pressure Pounding SLEEP	MISSED MEALS YES NO
PAIN LOCATION FRONT BACK LEFT RIGHT TOP		WEATHER TEMP °	STRESS YES NO
		LIGHTS YES NO SOUNDS YES NO	SMELLS YES NO

FOODS CONSUMED (within last 24 hours)	PRODROME (1-2 hours before headache)	SYMPTOMS	AURA (20-30 mins before)
☐ Alcohol	☐ Excessive Thirst	☐ Distorted Vision	☐ Black Spots
☐ Artificial Sweetener	☐ Excessive Yawning	☐ Dizziness	☐ Flashing Lights
☐ Beans	☐ Face Sensitivity	☐ Irritability	☐ Lack of Vision
☐ Caffeine	☐ Irritability	☐ Light-headedness	☐ Numbness FACE ARM LEG
☐ Cheese	☐ Light Sensitivity	☐ Light Sensitivity	☐ Zig Zag Lines
☐ Chocolate	☐ Neck Tightness	☐ Malaise	☐
☐ Fermented Foods	☐ Unexplained Fatigue	☐ Nasal Congestion	☐
☐ MSG	☐ Visual Disturbances	☐ Nausea/Vomiting	TRIGGER & SYMPTOM NOTES
☐ Non Friendly Fruits	☐	☐ Sound Sensitivity	
☐ Nuts	☐	☐ Tender Scalp	
☐ Processed Meats	☐	☐	
☐	☐	☐	
☐	☐	☐	
☐	☐		

REMEDIES

(NATURAL)		(OTC- COUNTER MEDS)	(Rx - PREVENTIVE)	(Rx - RELIEF)	(SUPPLEMENTS)
☐ Acupuncture	☐ Ice Pack	☐ Excedrin	☐ Amitriptyline	☐ Naproxin	☐ B2
☐ Acupressure	☐ Massage	☐ Ibuprofen	☐ Atenolol	☐ Nurtec	☐ Butterbur
☐ Caffeine	☐ Relaxation	☐ Tylenol	☐ Gabapentin	☐ Sumatriptan	☐ Feverfew
☐ Dark Room	☐ Silence	☐	☐ Nurtriptyline	☐ Rizatriptan	☐ Magnesium
☐ Hot Compress	☐ Walk	☐	☐ Propranolol	☐ Ubrelvy	☐
☐ Hydration	☐	☐	☐ Topamax	☐	☐
☐	☐	☐	☐ Valproate	☐	☐
☐	☐	☐	☐	WITHIN 1 HR OF PAIN YES NO	PAIN RELIEF YES NO
☐	☐	☐	☐		

REMEDY NOTES

IMPACT ON DAILY ACTIVITIES

NONE | MILD | MODERATE | SEVERE

WWW.ONEMINUTEMIGRAINEDIARY.COM

One Minute MIGRAINE Diary

Date : ____________

Start Time : ____________ End Time : ____________ Duration : ____________

PAIN SCALE [1-10]

|-----|-----|-----|-----|-----|-----|-----|-----|-----|
1 2 3 4 5 6 7 8 9 10
MILD MODERATE SEVERE

MENSTRUAL PERIOD
YES NO

Birth Control Pills
YES NO

PAIN TYPE
Stabbing Burning Pulsating Shocking Pressure Pounding

SLEEP

WATER

MISSED MEALS
YES NO

PAIN LOCATION

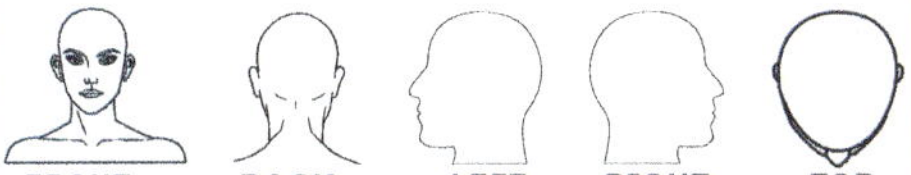

FRONT BACK LEFT RIGHT TOP

WEATHER
TEMP °

STRESS
YES NO

LIGHTS
YES NO

SOUNDS
YES NO

SMELLS
YES NO

FOODS CONSUMED (within last 24 hours)
- ☐ Alcohol
- ☐ Artificial Sweetener
- ☐ Beans
- ☐ Caffeine
- ☐ Cheese
- ☐ Chocolate
- ☐ Fermented Foods
- ☐ MSG
- ☐ Non Friendly Fruits
- ☐ Nuts
- ☐ Processed Meats
- ☐
- ☐
- ☐

PRODROME (1-2 hours before headache)
- ☐ Excessive Thirst
- ☐ Excessive Yawning
- ☐ Face Sensitivity
- ☐ Irritability
- ☐ Light Sensitivity
- ☐ Neck Tightness
- ☐ Unexplained Fatigue
- ☐ Visual Disturbances
- ☐
- ☐
- ☐
- ☐
- ☐

SYMPTOMS
- ☐ Distorted Vision
- ☐ Dizziness
- ☐ Irritability
- ☐ Light-headedness
- ☐ Light Sensitivity
- ☐ Malaise
- ☐ Nasal Congestion
- ☐ Nausea/Vomiting
- ☐ Sound Sensitivity
- ☐ Tender Scalp
- ☐
- ☐
- ☐

AURA (20-30 mins before)
- ☐ Black Spots
- ☐ Flashing Lights
- ☐ Lack of Vision
- ☐ Numbness FACE ARM LEG
- ☐ Zig Zag Lines
- ☐
- ☐

TRIGGER & SYMPTOM NOTES

REMEDIES

(NATURAL)
- ☐ Acupuncture
- ☐ Acupressure
- ☐ Caffeine
- ☐ Dark Room
- ☐ Hot Compress
- ☐ Hydration
- ☐
- ☐
- ☐
- ☐ Ice Pack
- ☐ Massage
- ☐ Relaxation
- ☐ Silence
- ☐ Walk
- ☐
- ☐
- ☐
- ☐

(OTC- COUNTER MEDS)
- ☐ Excedrin
- ☐ Ibuprofen
- ☐ Tylenol
- ☐
- ☐
- ☐
- ☐
- ☐
- ☐

(Rx - PREVENTIVE)
- ☐ Amitriptyline
- ☐ Atenolol
- ☐ Gabapentin
- ☐ Nurtriptyline
- ☐ Propranolol
- ☐ Topamax
- ☐ Valproate
- ☐
- ☐

(Rx - RELIEF)
- ☐ Naproxin
- ☐ Nurtec
- ☐ Sumatriptan
- ☐ Rizatriptan
- ☐ Ubrelvy
- ☐
- ☐

(SUPPLEMENTS)
- ☐ B2
- ☐ Butterbur
- ☐ Feverfew
- ☐ Magnesium
- ☐
- ☐
- ☐

WITHIN 1 HR OF PAIN YES NO PAIN RELIEF YES NO

REMEDY NOTES

IMPACT ON DAILY ACTIVITIES
NONE | MILD | MODERATE | SEVERE

WWW.ONEMINUTEMIGRAINEDIARY.COM

One Minute MIGRAINE Diary

Date : ____________________

Start Time : ______________ End Time : ____________ Duration : ______

PAIN SCALE [1-10]

1 2 3 4 5 6 7 8 9 10

MILD MODERATE SEVERE

MENSTRUAL PERIOD

YES NO

Birth Control Pills

YES NO

PAIN TYPE

Stabbing Burning Pulsating Shocking Pressure Pounding

SLEEP

WATER

MISSED MEALS

YES NO

PAIN LOCATION

FRONT BACK LEFT RIGHT TOP

WEATHER

TEMP °

STRESS

YES NO

LIGHTS

YES NO

SOUNDS

YES NO

SMELLS

YES NO

FOODS CONSUMED
(within last 24 hours)

- ☐ Alcohol
- ☐ Artificial Sweetener
- ☐ Beans
- ☐ Caffeine
- ☐ Cheese
- ☐ Chocolate
- ☐ Fermented Foods
- ☐ MSG
- ☐ Non Friendly Fruits
- ☐ Nuts
- ☐ Processed Meats
- ☐
- ☐
- ☐

PRODROME
(1-2 hours before headache)

- ☐ Excessive Thirst
- ☐ Excessive Yawning
- ☐ Face Sensitivity
- ☐ Irritability
- ☐ Light Sensitivity
- ☐ Neck Tightness
- ☐ Unexplained Fatigue
- ☐ Visual Disturbances
- ☐
- ☐
- ☐
- ☐
- ☐

SYMPTOMS

- ☐ Distorted Vision
- ☐ Dizziness
- ☐ Irritability
- ☐ Light-headedness
- ☐ Light Sensitivity
- ☐ Malaise
- ☐ Nasal Congestion
- ☐ Nausea/Vomiting
- ☐ Sound Sensitivity
- ☐ Tender Scalp
- ☐
- ☐
- ☐

AURA
(20-30 mins before)

- ☐ Black Spots
- ☐ Flashing Lights
- ☐ Lack of Vision
- ☐ Numbness FACE ARM LEG
- ☐ Zig Zag Lines
- ☐
- ☐

TRIGGER & SYMPTOM NOTES

REMEDIES

(NATURAL)

- ☐ Acupuncture
- ☐ Acupressure
- ☐ Caffeine
- ☐ Dark Room
- ☐ Hot Compress
- ☐ Hydration
- ☐
- ☐
- ☐
- ☐ Ice Pack
- ☐ Massage
- ☐ Relaxation
- ☐ Silence
- ☐ Walk
- ☐
- ☐
- ☐
- ☐

(OTC- COUNTER MEDS)

- ☐ Excedrin
- ☐ Ibuprofen
- ☐ Tylenol
- ☐
- ☐
- ☐
- ☐
- ☐
- ☐

(Rx - PREVENTIVE)

- ☐ Amitriptyline
- ☐ Atenolol
- ☐ Gabapentin
- ☐ Nurtriptyline
- ☐ Propranolol
- ☐ Topamax
- ☐ Valproate
- ☐
- ☐

(Rx - RELIEF)

- ☐ Naproxin
- ☐ Nurtec
- ☐ Sumatriptan
- ☐ Rizatriptan
- ☐ Ubrelvy
- ☐
- ☐

(SUPPLEMENTS)

- ☐ B2
- ☐ Butterbur
- ☐ Feverfew
- ☐ Magnesium
- ☐
- ☐
- ☐

WITHIN 1 HR OF PAIN YES NO

PAIN RELIEF YES NO

REMEDY NOTES

IMPACT ON DAILY ACTIVITIES

NONE | MILD | MODERATE | SEVERE

WWW.ONEMINUTEMIGRAINEDIARY.COM

One Minute MIGRAINE Diary

Date : ______________________

Start Time : ______________ End Time : ____________ Duration : ______

PAIN SCALE [1-10]

1 2 3 4 5 6 7 8 9 10

MILD MODERATE SEVERE

MENSTRUAL PERIOD

YES NO

Birth Control Pills

YES NO

PAIN TYPE

Stabbing Burning Pulsating Shocking Pressure Pounding

SLEEP

WATER

MISSED MEALS

YES NO

PAIN LOCATION

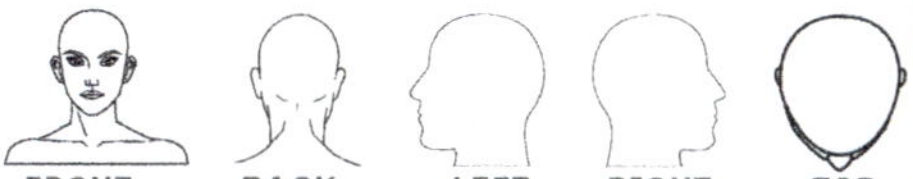

FRONT BACK LEFT RIGHT TOP

WEATHER

TEMP °

STRESS

YES NO

LIGHTS

YES NO

SOUNDS

YES NO

SMELLS

YES NO

FOODS CONSUMED
(within last 24 hours)

- ☐ Alcohol
- ☐ Artificial Sweetener
- ☐ Beans
- ☐ Caffeine
- ☐ Cheese
- ☐ Chocolate
- ☐ Fermented Foods
- ☐ MSG
- ☐ Non Friendly Fruits
- ☐ Nuts
- ☐ Processed Meats
- ☐
- ☐
- ☐

PRODROME
(1-2 hours before headache)

- ☐ Excessive Thirst
- ☐ Excessive Yawning
- ☐ Face Sensitivity
- ☐ Irritability
- ☐ Light Sensitivity
- ☐ Neck Tightness
- ☐ Unexplained Fatigue
- ☐ Visual Disturbances
- ☐
- ☐
- ☐
- ☐
- ☐

SYMPTOMS

- ☐ Distorted Vision
- ☐ Dizziness
- ☐ Irritability
- ☐ Light-headedness
- ☐ Light Sensitivity
- ☐ Malaise
- ☐ Nasal Congestion
- ☐ Nausea/Vomiting
- ☐ Sound Sensitivity
- ☐ Tender Scalp
- ☐
- ☐
- ☐

AURA
(20-30 mins before)

- ☐ Black Spots
- ☐ Flashing Lights
- ☐ Lack of Vision
- ☐ Numbness FACE ARM LEG
- ☐ Zig Zag Lines
- ☐
- ☐

TRIGGER & SYMPTOM NOTES

REMEDIES

(NATURAL)

- ☐ Acupuncture
- ☐ Acupressure
- ☐ Caffeine
- ☐ Dark Room
- ☐ Hot Compress
- ☐ Hydration
- ☐
- ☐
- ☐
- ☐ Ice Pack
- ☐ Massage
- ☐ Relaxation
- ☐ Silence
- ☐ Walk
- ☐
- ☐
- ☐
- ☐

(OTC- COUNTER MEDS)

- ☐ Excedrin
- ☐ Ibuprofen
- ☐ Tylenol
- ☐
- ☐
- ☐
- ☐
- ☐
- ☐

(Rx - PREVENTIVE)

- ☐ Amitriptyline
- ☐ Atenolol
- ☐ Gabapentin
- ☐ Nurtriptyline
- ☐ Propranolol
- ☐ Topamax
- ☐ Valproate
- ☐
- ☐

(Rx - RELIEF)

- ☐ Naproxin
- ☐ Nurtec
- ☐ Sumatriptan
- ☐ Rizatriptan
- ☐ Ubrelvy
- ☐
- ☐

(SUPPLEMENTS)

- ☐ B2
- ☐ Butterbur
- ☐ Feverfew
- ☐ Magnesium
- ☐
- ☐
- ☐

WITHIN 1 HR OF PAIN YES NO PAIN RELIEF YES NO

REMEDY NOTES

IMPACT ON DAILY ACTIVITIES

NONE | MILD | MODERATE | SEVERE

WWW.ONEMINUTEMIGRAINEDIARY.COM

One Minute MIGRAINE Diary

Date : ____________________

Start Time : ______________ End Time : ______________ Duration : ________

PAIN SCALE [1-10]

|-----|-----|-----|-----|-----|-----|-----|-----|-----|
1 2 3 4 5 6 7 8 9 10
MILD MODERATE SEVERE

MENSTRUAL PERIOD
YES NO

Birth Control Pills
YES NO

PAIN TYPE
Stabbing Burning Pulsating Shocking Pressure Pounding

SLEEP

WATER

MISSED MEALS
YES NO

PAIN LOCATION

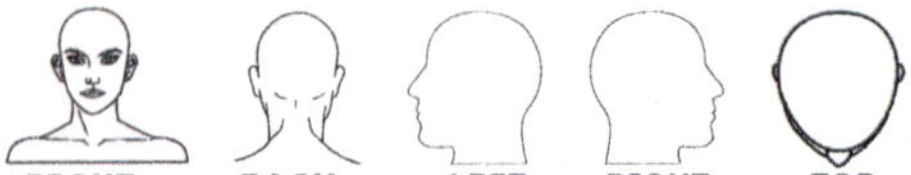

FRONT BACK LEFT RIGHT TOP

WEATHER
° TEMP

STRESS
YES NO

LIGHTS
YES NO

SOUNDS
YES NO

SMELLS
YES NO

FOODS CONSUMED (within last 24 hours)
- ☐ Alcohol
- ☐ Artificial Sweetener
- ☐ Beans
- ☐ Caffeine
- ☐ Cheese
- ☐ Chocolate
- ☐ Fermented Foods
- ☐ MSG
- ☐ Non Friendly Fruits
- ☐ Nuts
- ☐ Processed Meats
- ☐
- ☐
- ☐

PRODROME (1-2 hours before headache)
- ☐ Excessive Thirst
- ☐ Excessive Yawning
- ☐ Face Sensitivity
- ☐ Irritability
- ☐ Light Sensitivity
- ☐ Neck Tightness
- ☐ Unexplained Fatigue
- ☐ Visual Disturbances
- ☐
- ☐
- ☐
- ☐
- ☐

SYMPTOMS
- ☐ Distorted Vision
- ☐ Dizziness
- ☐ Irritability
- ☐ Light-headedness
- ☐ Light Sensitivity
- ☐ Malaise
- ☐ Nasal Congestion
- ☐ Nausea/Vomiting
- ☐ Sound Sensitivity
- ☐ Tender Scalp
- ☐
- ☐
- ☐

AURA (20-30 mins before)
- ☐ Black Spots
- ☐ Flashing Lights
- ☐ Lack of Vision
- ☐ Numbness FACE ARM LEG
- ☐ Zig Zag Lines
- ☐
- ☐

TRIGGER & SYMPTOM NOTES

REMEDIES

(NATURAL)
- ☐ Acupuncture
- ☐ Acupressure
- ☐ Caffeine
- ☐ Dark Room
- ☐ Hot Compress
- ☐ Hydration
- ☐
- ☐
- ☐
- ☐ Ice Pack
- ☐ Massage
- ☐ Relaxation
- ☐ Silence
- ☐ Walk
- ☐
- ☐
- ☐
- ☐

(OTC- COUNTER MEDS)
- ☐ Excedrin
- ☐ Ibuprofen
- ☐ Tylenol
- ☐
- ☐
- ☐
- ☐
- ☐
- ☐

(Rx - PREVENTIVE)
- ☐ Amitriptyline
- ☐ Atenolol
- ☐ Gabapentin
- ☐ Nurtriptyline
- ☐ Propranolol
- ☐ Topamax
- ☐ Valproate
- ☐
- ☐

(Rx - RELIEF)
- ☐ Naproxin
- ☐ Nurtec
- ☐ Sumatriptan
- ☐ Rizatriptan
- ☐ Ubrelvy
- ☐
- ☐

(SUPPLEMENTS)
- ☐ B2
- ☐ Butterbur
- ☐ Feverfew
- ☐ Magnesium
- ☐
- ☐
- ☐

WITHIN 1 HR OF PAIN YES NO PAIN RELIEF YES NO

REMEDY NOTES

IMPACT ON DAILY ACTIVITIES
NONE | MILD | MODERATE | SEVERE

WWW.ONEMINUTEMIGRAINEDIARY.COM

One Minute MIGRAINE Diary

Date : ____________________

Start Time : ____________ End Time : ____________ Duration : ________

PAIN SCALE [1-10]	MENSTRUAL PERIOD	PAIN TYPE	WATER
1 2 3 4 5 6 7 8 9 10 MILD MODERATE SEVERE	YES NO Birth Control Pills YES NO	Stabbing Burning Pulsating Shocking Pressure Pounding SLEEP	MISSED MEALS YES NO

PAIN LOCATION	WEATHER	STRESS
FRONT BACK LEFT RIGHT TOP	TEMP °	YES NO
	LIGHTS YES NO / SOUNDS YES NO	SMELLS YES NO

FOODS CONSUMED (within last 24 hours)	PRODROME (1-2 hours before headache)	SYMPTOMS	AURA (20-30 mins before)
☐ Alcohol	☐ Excessive Thirst	☐ Distorted Vision	☐ Black Spots
☐ Artificial Sweetener	☐ Excessive Yawning	☐ Dizziness	☐ Flashing Lights
☐ Beans	☐ Face Sensitivity	☐ Irritability	☐ Lack of Vision
☐ Caffeine	☐ Irritability	☐ Light-headedness	☐ Numbness FACE ARM LEG
☐ Cheese	☐ Light Sensitivity	☐ Light Sensitivity	☐ Zig Zag Lines
☐ Chocolate	☐ Neck Tightness	☐ Malaise	☐
☐ Fermented Foods	☐ Unexplained Fatigue	☐ Nasal Congestion	☐
☐ MSG	☐ Visual Disturbances	☐ Nausea/Vomiting	TRIGGER & SYMPTOM NOTES
☐ Non Friendly Fruits	☐	☐ Sound Sensitivity	
☐ Nuts	☐	☐ Tender Scalp	
☐ Processed Meats	☐	☐	
☐	☐	☐	
☐	☐	☐	
☐	☐		

REMEDIES

(NATURAL)		(OTC- COUNTER MEDS)	(Rx - PREVENTIVE)	(Rx - RELIEF)	(SUPPLEMENTS)
☐ Acupuncture	☐ Ice Pack	☐ Excedrin	☐ Amitriptyline	☐ Naproxin	☐ B2
☐ Acupressure	☐ Massage	☐ Ibuprofen	☐ Atenolol	☐ Nurtec	☐ Butterbur
☐ Caffeine	☐ Relaxation	☐ Tylenol	☐ Gabapentin	☐ Sumatriptan	☐ Feverfew
☐ Dark Room	☐ Silence	☐	☐ Nurtriptyline	☐ Rizatriptan	☐ Magnesium
☐ Hot Compress	☐ Walk	☐	☐ Propranolol	☐ Ubrelvy	☐
☐ Hydration	☐	☐	☐ Topamax	☐	☐
☐	☐	☐	☐ Valproate	☐	☐
☐	☐	☐	☐	WITHIN 1 HR OF PAIN YES NO	PAIN RELIEF YES NO
☐	☐	☐	☐		

REMEDY NOTES

IMPACT ON DAILY ACTIVITIES

NONE | MILD | MODERATE | SEVERE

WWW.ONEMINUTEMIGRAINEDIARY.COM

One Minute MIGRAINE Diary

Date : ____________________

Start Time : ______________ End Time : ______________ Duration : ________

PAIN SCALE [1-10]
1 2 3 4 5 6 7 8 9 10
MILD MODERATE SEVERE

MENSTRUAL PERIOD
YES NO
Birth Control Pills
YES NO

PAIN TYPE
Stabbing Burning Pulsating Shocking Pressure Pounding

SLEEP

WATER

MISSED MEALS
YES NO

PAIN LOCATION
FRONT BACK LEFT RIGHT TOP

WEATHER
TEMP °

STRESS
YES NO

LIGHTS
YES NO

SOUNDS
YES NO

SMELLS
YES NO

FOODS CONSUMED (within last 24 hours)
- ☐ Alcohol
- ☐ Artificial Sweetener
- ☐ Beans
- ☐ Caffeine
- ☐ Cheese
- ☐ Chocolate
- ☐ Fermented Foods
- ☐ MSG
- ☐ Non Friendly Fruits
- ☐ Nuts
- ☐ Processed Meats
- ☐
- ☐
- ☐

PRODROME (1-2 hours before headache)
- ☐ Excessive Thirst
- ☐ Excessive Yawning
- ☐ Face Sensitivity
- ☐ Irritability
- ☐ Light Sensitivity
- ☐ Neck Tightness
- ☐ Unexplained Fatigue
- ☐ Visual Disturbances
- ☐
- ☐
- ☐
- ☐
- ☐

SYMPTOMS
- ☐ Distorted Vision
- ☐ Dizziness
- ☐ Irritability
- ☐ Light-headedness
- ☐ Light Sensitivity
- ☐ Malaise
- ☐ Nasal Congestion
- ☐ Nausea/Vomiting
- ☐ Sound Sensitivity
- ☐ Tender Scalp
- ☐
- ☐
- ☐

AURA (20-30 mins before)
- ☐ Black Spots
- ☐ Flashing Lights
- ☐ Lack of Vision
- ☐ Numbness FACE ARM LEG
- ☐ Zig Zag Lines
- ☐
- ☐

TRIGGER & SYMPTOM NOTES

REMEDIES

(NATURAL)
- ☐ Acupuncture
- ☐ Acupressure
- ☐ Caffeine
- ☐ Dark Room
- ☐ Hot Compress
- ☐ Hydration
- ☐
- ☐
- ☐
- ☐ Ice Pack
- ☐ Massage
- ☐ Relaxation
- ☐ Silence
- ☐ Walk
- ☐
- ☐
- ☐
- ☐

(OTC- COUNTER MEDS)
- ☐ Excedrin
- ☐ Ibuprofen
- ☐ Tylenol
- ☐
- ☐
- ☐
- ☐
- ☐
- ☐

(Rx - PREVENTIVE)
- ☐ Amitriptyline
- ☐ Atenolol
- ☐ Gabapentin
- ☐ Nurtriptyline
- ☐ Propranolol
- ☐ Topamax
- ☐ Valproate
- ☐
- ☐

(Rx - RELIEF)
- ☐ Naproxin
- ☐ Nurtec
- ☐ Sumatriptan
- ☐ Rizatriptan
- ☐ Ubrelvy
- ☐
- ☐

(SUPPLEMENTS)
- ☐ B2
- ☐ Butterbur
- ☐ Feverfew
- ☐ Magnesium
- ☐
- ☐
- ☐

WITHIN 1 HR OF PAIN YES NO PAIN RELIEF YES NO

REMEDY NOTES

IMPACT ON DAILY ACTIVITIES
NONE | MILD | MODERATE | SEVERE

WWW.ONEMINUTEMIGRAINEDIARY.COM

One Minute MIGRAINE Diary

Date : ____________________

Start Time : ____________________ End Time : ____________ Duration : ________

PAIN SCALE [1-10]	MENSTRUAL PERIOD	PAIN TYPE	WATER
1 2 3 4 5 6 7 8 9 10 MILD MODERATE SEVERE	YES NO Birth Control Pills YES NO	Stabbing Burning Pulsating Shocking Pressure Pounding **SLEEP**	**MISSED MEALS** YES NO
PAIN LOCATION FRONT BACK LEFT RIGHT TOP		**WEATHER** TEMP	**STRESS** YES NO
		LIGHTS YES NO **SOUNDS** YES NO	**SMELLS** YES NO

FOODS CONSUMED (within last 24 hours)	PRODROME (1-2 hours before headache)	SYMPTOMS	AURA (20-30 mins before)
☐ Alcohol	☐ Excessive Thirst	☐ Distorted Vision	☐ Black Spots
☐ Artificial Sweetener	☐ Excessive Yawning	☐ Dizziness	☐ Flashing Lights
☐ Beans	☐ Face Sensitivity	☐ Irritability	☐ Lack of Vision
☐ Caffeine	☐ Irritability	☐ Light-headedness	☐ Numbness FACE ARM LEG
☐ Cheese	☐ Light Sensitivity	☐ Light Sensitivity	☐ Zig Zag Lines
☐ Chocolate	☐ Neck Tightness	☐ Malaise	☐
☐ Fermented Foods	☐ Unexplained Fatigue	☐ Nasal Congestion	☐
☐ MSG	☐ Visual Disturbances	☐ Nausea/Vomiting	**TRIGGER & SYMPTOM NOTES**
☐ Non Friendly Fruits	☐	☐ Sound Sensitivity	
☐ Nuts	☐	☐ Tender Scalp	
☐ Processed Meats	☐	☐	
☐	☐	☐	
☐	☐	☐	
☐			

REMEDIES

(NATURAL)		(OTC- COUNTER MEDS)	(Rx - PREVENTIVE)	(Rx - RELIEF)	(SUPPLEMENTS)
☐ Acupuncture	☐ Ice Pack	☐ Excedrin	☐ Amitriptyline	☐ Naproxin	☐ B2
☐ Acupressure	☐ Massage	☐ Ibuprofen	☐ Atenolol	☐ Nurtec	☐ Butterbur
☐ Caffeine	☐ Relaxation	☐ Tylenol	☐ Gabapentin	☐ Sumatriptan	☐ Feverfew
☐ Dark Room	☐ Silence	☐	☐ Nurtriptyline	☐ Rizatriptan	☐ Magnesium
☐ Hot Compress	☐ Walk	☐	☐ Propranolol	☐ Ubrelvy	☐
☐ Hydration	☐	☐	☐ Topamax	☐	☐
☐	☐	☐	☐ Valproate	☐	☐
☐	☐	☐	☐	WITHIN 1 HR OF PAIN YES NO	PAIN RELIEF YES NO
☐	☐	☐	☐		

REMEDY NOTES

IMPACT ON DAILY ACTIVITIES

NONE | MILD | MODERATE | SEVERE

WWW.ONEMINUTEMIGRAINEDIARY.COM

One Minute MIGRAINE Diary

Date : ______________________

Start Time : ________________ End Time : ______________ Duration : ________

PAIN SCALE [1-10]	MENSTRUAL PERIOD	PAIN TYPE	WATER
1 2 3 4 5 6 7 8 9 10 MILD MODERATE SEVERE	YES NO Birth Control Pills YES NO	Stabbing Burning Pulsating Shocking Pressure Pounding **SLEEP**	**MISSED MEALS** YES NO

PAIN LOCATION

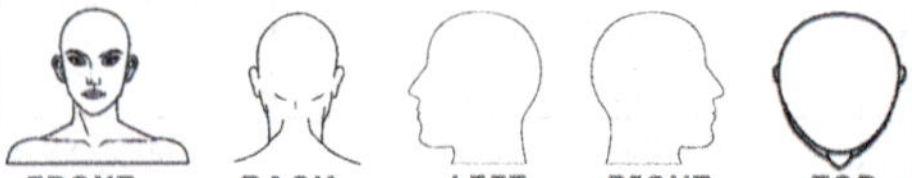

FRONT BACK LEFT RIGHT TOP

WEATHER

TEMP °

LIGHTS YES NO

SOUNDS YES NO

STRESS YES NO

SMELLS YES NO

FOODS CONSUMED (within last 24 hours)	PRODROME (1-2 hours before headache)	SYMPTOMS	AURA (20-30 mins before)
☐ Alcohol	☐ Excessive Thirst	☐ Distorted Vision	☐ Black Spots
☐ Artificial Sweetener	☐ Excessive Yawning	☐ Dizziness	☐ Flashing Lights
☐ Beans	☐ Face Sensitivity	☐ Irritability	☐ Lack of Vision
☐ Caffeine	☐ Irritability	☐ Light-headedness	☐ Numbness FACE ARM LEG
☐ Cheese	☐ Light Sensitivity	☐ Light Sensitivity	☐ Zig Zag Lines
☐ Chocolate	☐ Neck Tightness	☐ Malaise	☐
☐ Fermented Foods	☐ Unexplained Fatigue	☐ Nasal Congestion	☐
☐ MSG	☐ Visual Disturbances	☐ Nausea/Vomiting	**TRIGGER & SYMPTOM NOTES**
☐ Non Friendly Fruits	☐	☐ Sound Sensitivity	
☐ Nuts	☐	☐ Tender Scalp	
☐ Processed Meats	☐	☐	
☐	☐	☐	
☐	☐	☐	
☐			

REMEDIES

(NATURAL)		(OTC- COUNTER MEDS)	(Rx - PREVENTIVE)	(Rx - RELIEF)	(SUPPLEMENTS)
☐ Acupuncture	☐ Ice Pack	☐ Excedrin	☐ Amitriptyline	☐ Naproxin	☐ B2
☐ Acupressure	☐ Massage	☐ Ibuprofen	☐ Atenolol	☐ Nurtec	☐ Butterbur
☐ Caffeine	☐ Relaxation	☐ Tylenol	☐ Gabapentin	☐ Sumatriptan	☐ Feverfew
☐ Dark Room	☐ Silence	☐	☐ Nurtriptyline	☐ Rizatriptan	☐ Magnesium
☐ Hot Compress	☐ Walk	☐	☐ Propranolol	☐ Ubrelvy	☐
☐ Hydration	☐	☐	☐ Topamax	☐	☐
☐	☐	☐	☐ Valproate	☐	☐
☐	☐	☐	☐	WITHIN 1 HR OF PAIN YES NO	PAIN RELIEF YES NO
☐	☐	☐	☐		

REMEDY NOTES

IMPACT ON DAILY ACTIVITIES

NONE | MILD | MODERATE | SEVERE

WWW.ONEMINUTEMIGRAINEDIARY.COM

One Minute MIGRAINE Diary

Date :

Start Time : End Time : Duration :

PAIN SCALE [1-10]

1 2 3 4 5 6 7 8 9 10

MILD MODERATE SEVERE

MENSTRUAL PERIOD YES NO

Birth Control Pills YES NO

PAIN TYPE

Stabbing Burning Pulsating Shocking Pressure Pounding

SLEEP

WATER

MISSED MEALS YES NO

PAIN LOCATION

FRONT BACK LEFT RIGHT TOP

WEATHER

TEMP °

STRESS YES NO

LIGHTS YES NO

SOUNDS YES NO

SMELLS YES NO

FOODS CONSUMED (within last 24 hours)

- ☐ Alcohol
- ☐ Artificial Sweetener
- ☐ Beans
- ☐ Caffeine
- ☐ Cheese
- ☐ Chocolate
- ☐ Fermented Foods
- ☐ MSG
- ☐ Non Friendly Fruits
- ☐ Nuts
- ☐ Processed Meats
- ☐
- ☐
- ☐

PRODROME (1-2 hours before headache)

- ☐ Excessive Thirst
- ☐ Excessive Yawning
- ☐ Face Sensitivity
- ☐ Irritability
- ☐ Light Sensitivity
- ☐ Neck Tightness
- ☐ Unexplained Fatigue
- ☐ Visual Disturbances
- ☐
- ☐
- ☐
- ☐
- ☐

SYMPTOMS

- ☐ Distorted Vision
- ☐ Dizziness
- ☐ Irritability
- ☐ Light-headedness
- ☐ Light Sensitivity
- ☐ Malaise
- ☐ Nasal Congestion
- ☐ Nausea/Vomiting
- ☐ Sound Sensitivity
- ☐ Tender Scalp
- ☐
- ☐
- ☐

AURA (20-30 mins before)

- ☐ Black Spots
- ☐ Flashing Lights
- ☐ Lack of Vision
- ☐ Numbness FACE ARM LEG
- ☐ Zig Zag Lines
- ☐
- ☐

TRIGGER & SYMPTOM NOTES

REMEDIES

(NATURAL)

- ☐ Acupuncture
- ☐ Acupressure
- ☐ Caffeine
- ☐ Dark Room
- ☐ Hot Compress
- ☐ Hydration
- ☐
- ☐
- ☐
- ☐ Ice Pack
- ☐ Massage
- ☐ Relaxation
- ☐ Silence
- ☐ Walk
- ☐
- ☐
- ☐
- ☐

(OTC- COUNTER MEDS)

- ☐ Excedrin
- ☐ Ibuprofen
- ☐ Tylenol
- ☐
- ☐
- ☐
- ☐
- ☐
- ☐

(Rx - PREVENTIVE)

- ☐ Amitriptyline
- ☐ Atenolol
- ☐ Gabapentin
- ☐ Nurtriptyline
- ☐ Propranolol
- ☐ Topamax
- ☐ Valproate
- ☐
- ☐

(Rx - RELIEF)

- ☐ Naproxin
- ☐ Nurtec
- ☐ Sumatriptan
- ☐ Rizatriptan
- ☐ Ubrelvy
- ☐
- ☐

(SUPPLEMENTS)

- ☐ B2
- ☐ Butterbur
- ☐ Feverfew
- ☐ Magnesium
- ☐
- ☐
- ☐

WITHIN 1 HR OF PAIN YES NO

PAIN RELIEF YES NO

REMEDY NOTES

IMPACT ON DAILY ACTIVITIES

NONE | MILD | MODERATE | SEVERE

WWW.ONEMINUTEMIGRAINEDIARY.COM

One Minute MIGRAINE Diary

Date : ____________________

Start Time : ____________ End Time : ____________ Duration : ________

PAIN SCALE [1-10]	MENSTRUAL PERIOD	PAIN TYPE	WATER
1 2 3 4 5 6 7 8 9 10 MILD MODERATE SEVERE	YES NO Birth Control Pills YES NO	Stabbing Burning Pulsating Shocking Pressure Pounding SLEEP	MISSED MEALS YES NO

PAIN LOCATION	WEATHER	STRESS
FRONT BACK LEFT RIGHT TOP	TEMP °	YES NO
	LIGHTS YES NO · SOUNDS YES NO	SMELLS YES NO

FOODS CONSUMED (within last 24 hours)	PRODROME (1-2 hours before headache)	SYMPTOMS	AURA (20-30 mins before)
☐ Alcohol	☐ Excessive Thirst	☐ Distorted Vision	☐ Black Spots
☐ Artificial Sweetener	☐ Excessive Yawning	☐ Dizziness	☐ Flashing Lights
☐ Beans	☐ Face Sensitivity	☐ Irritability	☐ Lack of Vision
☐ Caffeine	☐ Irritability	☐ Light-headedness	☐ Numbness FACE ARM LEG
☐ Cheese	☐ Light Sensitivity	☐ Light Sensitivity	☐ Zig Zag Lines
☐ Chocolate	☐ Neck Tightness	☐ Malaise	☐
☐ Fermented Foods	☐ Unexplained Fatigue	☐ Nasal Congestion	☐
☐ MSG	☐ Visual Disturbances	☐ Nausea/Vomiting	TRIGGER & SYMPTOM NOTES
☐ Non Friendly Fruits	☐	☐ Sound Sensitivity	
☐ Nuts	☐	☐ Tender Scalp	
☐ Processed Meats	☐	☐	
☐	☐	☐	
☐	☐	☐	
☐			

REMEDIES

(NATURAL)		(OTC- COUNTER MEDS)	(Rx - PREVENTIVE)	(Rx - RELIEF)	(SUPPLEMENTS)
☐ Acupuncture	☐ Ice Pack	☐ Excedrin	☐ Amitriptyline	☐ Naproxin	☐ B2
☐ Acupressure	☐ Massage	☐ Ibuprofen	☐ Atenolol	☐ Nurtec	☐ Butterbur
☐ Caffeine	☐ Relaxation	☐ Tylenol	☐ Gabapentin	☐ Sumatriptan	☐ Feverfew
☐ Dark Room	☐ Silence	☐	☐ Nurtriptyline	☐ Rizatriptan	☐ Magnesium
☐ Hot Compress	☐ Walk	☐	☐ Propranolol	☐ Ubrelvy	☐
☐ Hydration	☐	☐	☐ Topamax	☐	☐
☐	☐	☐	☐ Valproate	☐	☐
☐	☐	☐	☐	WITHIN 1 HR OF PAIN YES NO	PAIN RELIEF YES NO
☐	☐	☐	☐		

REMEDY NOTES

IMPACT ON DAILY ACTIVITIES

NONE | MILD | MODERATE | SEVERE

WWW.ONEMINUTEMIGRAINEDIARY.COM

One Minute MIGRAINE Diary

Date : ____________

Start Time : ____________ End Time : ____________ Duration : ________

PAIN SCALE [1-10]	MENSTRUAL PERIOD	PAIN TYPE	WATER
1 2 3 4 5 6 7 8 9 10 MILD MODERATE SEVERE	YES NO Birth Control Pills YES NO	Stabbing Burning Pulsating Shocking Pressure Pounding SLEEP	MISSED MEALS YES NO

PAIN LOCATION	WEATHER	STRESS
FRONT BACK LEFT RIGHT TOP	TEMP	YES NO
	LIGHTS YES NO / SOUNDS YES NO	SMELLS YES NO

FOODS CONSUMED (within last 24 hours)	PRODROME (1-2 hours before headache)	SYMPTOMS	AURA (20-30 mins before)
☐ Alcohol	☐ Excessive Thirst	☐ Distorted Vision	☐ Black Spots
☐ Artificial Sweetener	☐ Excessive Yawning	☐ Dizziness	☐ Flashing Lights
☐ Beans	☐ Face Sensitivity	☐ Irritability	☐ Lack of Vision
☐ Caffeine	☐ Irritability	☐ Light-headedness	☐ Numbness FACE ARM LEG
☐ Cheese	☐ Light Sensitivity	☐ Light Sensitivity	☐ Zig Zag Lines
☐ Chocolate	☐ Neck Tightness	☐ Malaise	☐
☐ Fermented Foods	☐ Unexplained Fatigue	☐ Nasal Congestion	☐
☐ MSG	☐ Visual Disturbances	☐ Nausea/Vomiting	TRIGGER & SYMPTOM NOTES
☐ Non Friendly Fruits	☐	☐ Sound Sensitivity	
☐ Nuts	☐	☐ Tender Scalp	
☐ Processed Meats	☐	☐	
☐	☐	☐	
☐	☐	☐	
☐	☐		

REMEDIES

(NATURAL)		(OTC- COUNTER MEDS)	(Rx - PREVENTIVE)	(Rx - RELIEF)	(SUPPLEMENTS)
☐ Acupuncture	☐ Ice Pack	☐ Excedrin	☐ Amitriptyline	☐ Naproxin	☐ B2
☐ Acupressure	☐ Massage	☐ Ibuprofen	☐ Atenolol	☐ Nurtec	☐ Butterbur
☐ Caffeine	☐ Relaxation	☐ Tylenol	☐ Gabapentin	☐ Sumatriptan	☐ Feverfew
☐ Dark Room	☐ Silence	☐	☐ Nurtriptyline	☐ Rizatriptan	☐ Magnesium
☐ Hot Compress	☐ Walk	☐	☐ Propranolol	☐ Ubrelvy	☐
☐ Hydration	☐	☐	☐ Topamax	☐	☐
☐	☐	☐	☐ Valproate	☐	☐
☐	☐	☐	☐	WITHIN 1 HR OF PAIN YES NO	PAIN RELIEF YES NO
☐	☐	☐	☐		

REMEDY NOTES

IMPACT ON DAILY ACTIVITIES

NONE | MILD | MODERATE | SEVERE

WWW.ONEMINUTEMIGRAINEDIARY.COM

One Minute MIGRAINE Diary

Date : ______________________

Start Time : ______________ End Time : ______________ Duration : __________

PAIN SCALE [1-10]

1 2 3 4 5 6 7 8 9 10

MILD MODERATE SEVERE

MENSTRUAL PERIOD

YES NO

Birth Control Pills

YES NO

PAIN TYPE

Stabbing Burning Pulsating Shocking Pressure Pounding

SLEEP

WATER

MISSED MEALS

YES NO

PAIN LOCATION

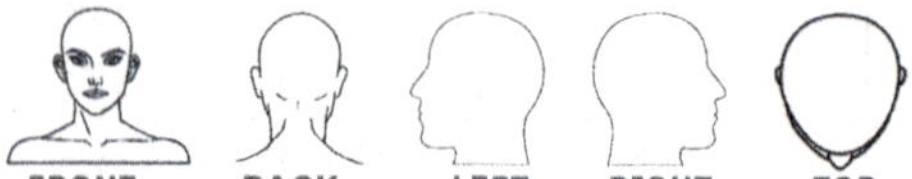

FRONT BACK LEFT RIGHT TOP

WEATHER

TEMP °

STRESS

YES NO

LIGHTS

YES NO

SOUNDS

YES NO

SMELLS

YES NO

FOODS CONSUMED (within last 24 hours)

- ☐ Alcohol
- ☐ Artificial Sweetener
- ☐ Beans
- ☐ Caffeine
- ☐ Cheese
- ☐ Chocolate
- ☐ Fermented Foods
- ☐ MSG
- ☐ Non Friendly Fruits
- ☐ Nuts
- ☐ Processed Meats
- ☐
- ☐
- ☐

PRODROME (1-2 hours before headache)

- ☐ Excessive Thirst
- ☐ Excessive Yawning
- ☐ Face Sensitivity
- ☐ Irritability
- ☐ Light Sensitivity
- ☐ Neck Tightness
- ☐ Unexplained Fatigue
- ☐ Visual Disturbances
- ☐
- ☐
- ☐
- ☐
- ☐

SYMPTOMS

- ☐ Distorted Vision
- ☐ Dizziness
- ☐ Irritability
- ☐ Light-headedness
- ☐ Light Sensitivity
- ☐ Malaise
- ☐ Nasal Congestion
- ☐ Nausea/Vomiting
- ☐ Sound Sensitivity
- ☐ Tender Scalp
- ☐
- ☐
- ☐

AURA (20-30 mins before)

- ☐ Black Spots
- ☐ Flashing Lights
- ☐ Lack of Vision
- ☐ Numbness FACE ARM LEG
- ☐ Zig Zag Lines
- ☐
- ☐

TRIGGER & SYMPTOM NOTES

REMEDIES

(NATURAL)

- ☐ Acupuncture
- ☐ Acupressure
- ☐ Caffeine
- ☐ Dark Room
- ☐ Hot Compress
- ☐ Hydration
- ☐
- ☐
- ☐
- ☐ Ice Pack
- ☐ Massage
- ☐ Relaxation
- ☐ Silence
- ☐ Walk
- ☐
- ☐
- ☐
- ☐

(OTC- COUNTER MEDS)

- ☐ Excedrin
- ☐ Ibuprofen
- ☐ Tylenol
- ☐
- ☐
- ☐
- ☐
- ☐
- ☐

(Rx - PREVENTIVE)

- ☐ Amitriptyline
- ☐ Atenolol
- ☐ Gabapentin
- ☐ Nurtriptyline
- ☐ Propranolol
- ☐ Topamax
- ☐ Valproate
- ☐
- ☐

(Rx - RELIEF)

- ☐ Naproxin
- ☐ Nurtec
- ☐ Sumatriptan
- ☐ Rizatriptan
- ☐ Ubrelvy
- ☐
- ☐

(SUPPLEMENTS)

- ☐ B2
- ☐ Butterbur
- ☐ Feverfew
- ☐ Magnesium
- ☐
- ☐
- ☐

WITHIN 1 HR OF PAIN YES NO

PAIN RELIEF YES NO

REMEDY NOTES

IMPACT ON DAILY ACTIVITIES

NONE | MILD | MODERATE | SEVERE

WWW.ONEMINUTEMIGRAINEDIARY.COM

One Minute MIGRAINE Diary

Date : ______________

Start Time : ______________ End Time : ______________ Duration : ________

PAIN SCALE [1-10]	MENSTRUAL PERIOD	PAIN TYPE	WATER
1 2 3 4 5 6 7 8 9 10 MILD MODERATE SEVERE	YES NO Birth Control Pills YES NO	Stabbing Burning Pulsating Shocking Pressure Pounding SLEEP	MISSED MEALS YES NO

PAIN LOCATION

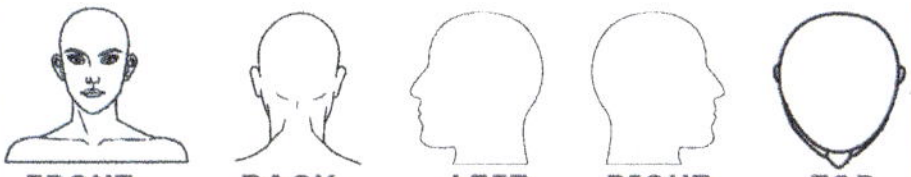

FRONT BACK LEFT RIGHT TOP

WEATHER

TEMP °

LIGHTS YES NO

SOUNDS YES NO

STRESS YES NO

SMELLS YES NO

FOODS CONSUMED (within last 24 hours)	PRODROME (1-2 hours before headache)	SYMPTOMS	AURA (20-30 mins before)
☐ Alcohol	☐ Excessive Thirst	☐ Distorted Vision	☐ Black Spots
☐ Artificial Sweetener	☐ Excessive Yawning	☐ Dizziness	☐ Flashing Lights
☐ Beans	☐ Face Sensitivity	☐ Irritability	☐ Lack of Vision
☐ Caffeine	☐ Irritability	☐ Light-headedness	☐ Numbness FACE ARM LEG
☐ Cheese	☐ Light Sensitivity	☐ Light Sensitivity	☐ Zig Zag Lines
☐ Chocolate	☐ Neck Tightness	☐ Malaise	☐
☐ Fermented Foods	☐ Unexplained Fatigue	☐ Nasal Congestion	☐
☐ MSG	☐ Visual Disturbances	☐ Nausea/Vomiting	TRIGGER & SYMPTOM NOTES
☐ Non Friendly Fruits	☐	☐ Sound Sensitivity	
☐ Nuts	☐	☐ Tender Scalp	
☐ Processed Meats	☐	☐	
☐	☐	☐	
☐	☐	☐	
☐	☐		

REMEDIES

(NATURAL)		(OTC- COUNTER MEDS)	(Rx - PREVENTIVE)	(Rx - RELIEF)	(SUPPLEMENTS)
☐ Acupuncture	☐ Ice Pack	☐ Excedrin	☐ Amitriptyline	☐ Naproxin	☐ B2
☐ Acupressure	☐ Massage	☐ Ibuprofen	☐ Atenolol	☐ Nurtec	☐ Butterbur
☐ Caffeine	☐ Relaxation	☐ Tylenol	☐ Gabapentin	☐ Sumatriptan	☐ Feverfew
☐ Dark Room	☐ Silence	☐	☐ Nurtriptyline	☐ Rizatriptan	☐ Magnesium
☐ Hot Compress	☐ Walk	☐	☐ Propranolol	☐ Ubrelvy	☐
☐ Hydration	☐	☐	☐ Topamax	☐	☐
☐	☐	☐	☐ Valproate	☐	☐
☐	☐	☐	☐	WITHIN 1 HR OF PAIN YES NO	PAIN RELIEF YES NO
☐	☐	☐	☐		

REMEDY NOTES

IMPACT ON DAILY ACTIVITIES

NONE | MILD | MODERATE | SEVERE

WWW.ONEMINUTEMIGRAINEDIARY.COM

One Minute MIGRAINE Diary

Date : ____________________

Start Time : ______________ End Time : ______________ Duration : ________

PAIN SCALE [1-10]	MENSTRUAL PERIOD	PAIN TYPE	WATER
1 2 3 4 5 6 7 8 9 10 MILD MODERATE SEVERE	YES NO Birth Control Pills YES NO	Stabbing Burning Pulsating Shocking Pressure Pounding SLEEP	MISSED MEALS YES NO

PAIN LOCATION

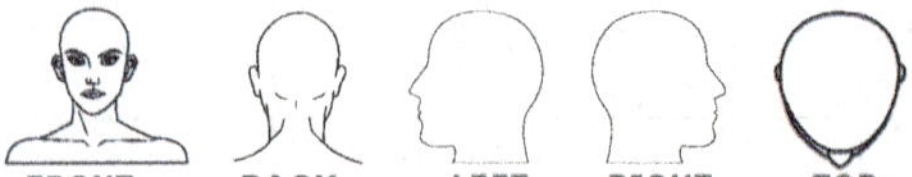

FRONT BACK LEFT RIGHT TOP

WEATHER

TEMP °

LIGHTS YES NO

SOUNDS YES NO

STRESS YES NO

SMELLS YES NO

FOODS CONSUMED (within last 24 hours)	PRODROME (1-2 hours before headache)	SYMPTOMS	AURA (20-30 mins before)
☐ Alcohol	☐ Excessive Thirst	☐ Distorted Vision	☐ Black Spots
☐ Artificial Sweetener	☐ Excessive Yawning	☐ Dizziness	☐ Flashing Lights
☐ Beans	☐ Face Sensitivity	☐ Irritability	☐ Lack of Vision
☐ Caffeine	☐ Irritability	☐ Light-headedness	☐ Numbness FACE ARM LEG
☐ Cheese	☐ Light Sensitivity	☐ Light Sensitivity	☐ Zig Zag Lines
☐ Chocolate	☐ Neck Tightness	☐ Malaise	☐
☐ Fermented Foods	☐ Unexplained Fatigue	☐ Nasal Congestion	☐
☐ MSG	☐ Visual Disturbances	☐ Nausea/Vomiting	TRIGGER & SYMPTOM NOTES
☐ Non Friendly Fruits	☐	☐ Sound Sensitivity	
☐ Nuts	☐	☐ Tender Scalp	
☐ Processed Meats	☐	☐	
☐	☐	☐	
☐	☐	☐	
☐			

REMEDIES

(NATURAL)		(OTC- COUNTER MEDS)	(Rx - PREVENTIVE)	(Rx - RELIEF)	(SUPPLEMENTS)
☐ Acupuncture	☐ Ice Pack	☐ Excedrin	☐ Amitriptyline	☐ Naproxin	☐ B2
☐ Acupressure	☐ Massage	☐ Ibuprofen	☐ Atenolol	☐ Nurtec	☐ Butterbur
☐ Caffeine	☐ Relaxation	☐ Tylenol	☐ Gabapentin	☐ Sumatriptan	☐ Feverfew
☐ Dark Room	☐ Silence	☐	☐ Nurtriptyline	☐ Rizatriptan	☐ Magnesium
☐ Hot Compress	☐ Walk	☐	☐ Propranolol	☐ Ubrelvy	☐
☐ Hydration	☐	☐	☐ Topamax	☐	☐
☐	☐	☐	☐ Valproate	☐	☐
☐	☐	☐	☐	WITHIN 1 HR OF PAIN YES NO	PAIN RELIEF YES NO
☐	☐	☐	☐		

REMEDY NOTES

IMPACT ON DAILY ACTIVITIES

NONE | MILD | MODERATE | SEVERE

WWW.ONEMINUTEMIGRAINEDIARY.COM

One Minute MIGRAINE Diary

Date : ______________

Start Time : ______________ End Time : ______________ Duration : ______

PAIN SCALE [1-10]

1 2 3 4 5 6 7 8 9 10

MILD MODERATE SEVERE

MENSTRUAL PERIOD

YES NO

Birth Control Pills

YES NO

PAIN TYPE

Stabbing Burning Pulsating Shocking Pressure Pounding

SLEEP

WATER

MISSED MEALS

YES NO

PAIN LOCATION

FRONT BACK LEFT RIGHT TOP

WEATHER

TEMP °

STRESS

YES NO

LIGHTS

YES NO

SOUNDS

YES NO

SMELLS

YES NO

FOODS CONSUMED (within last 24 hours)

- ☐ Alcohol
- ☐ Artificial Sweetener
- ☐ Beans
- ☐ Caffeine
- ☐ Cheese
- ☐ Chocolate
- ☐ Fermented Foods
- ☐ MSG
- ☐ Non Friendly Fruits
- ☐ Nuts
- ☐ Processed Meats
- ☐
- ☐
- ☐

PRODROME (1-2 hours before headache)

- ☐ Excessive Thirst
- ☐ Excessive Yawning
- ☐ Face Sensitivity
- ☐ Irritability
- ☐ Light Sensitivity
- ☐ Neck Tightness
- ☐ Unexplained Fatigue
- ☐ Visual Disturbances
- ☐
- ☐
- ☐
- ☐
- ☐

SYMPTOMS

- ☐ Distorted Vision
- ☐ Dizziness
- ☐ Irritability
- ☐ Light-headedness
- ☐ Light Sensitivity
- ☐ Malaise
- ☐ Nasal Congestion
- ☐ Nausea/Vomiting
- ☐ Sound Sensitivity
- ☐ Tender Scalp
- ☐
- ☐
- ☐

AURA (20-30 mins before)

- ☐ Black Spots
- ☐ Flashing Lights
- ☐ Lack of Vision
- ☐ Numbness FACE ARM LEG
- ☐ Zig Zag Lines
- ☐
- ☐

TRIGGER & SYMPTOM NOTES

REMEDIES

(NATURAL)

- ☐ Acupuncture
- ☐ Acupressure
- ☐ Caffeine
- ☐ Dark Room
- ☐ Hot Compress
- ☐ Hydration
- ☐
- ☐
- ☐
- ☐ Ice Pack
- ☐ Massage
- ☐ Relaxation
- ☐ Silence
- ☐ Walk
- ☐
- ☐
- ☐
- ☐

(OTC- COUNTER MEDS)

- ☐ Excedrin
- ☐ Ibuprofen
- ☐ Tylenol
- ☐
- ☐
- ☐
- ☐
- ☐
- ☐

(Rx - PREVENTIVE)

- ☐ Amitriptyline
- ☐ Atenolol
- ☐ Gabapentin
- ☐ Nurtriptyline
- ☐ Propranolol
- ☐ Topamax
- ☐ Valproate
- ☐
- ☐

(Rx - RELIEF)

- ☐ Naproxin
- ☐ Nurtec
- ☐ Sumatriptan
- ☐ Rizatriptan
- ☐ Ubrelvy
- ☐
- ☐

(SUPPLEMENTS)

- ☐ B2
- ☐ Butterbur
- ☐ Feverfew
- ☐ Magnesium
- ☐
- ☐
- ☐

WITHIN 1 HR OF PAIN YES NO PAIN RELIEF YES NO

REMEDY NOTES

IMPACT ON DAILY ACTIVITIES

NONE | MILD | MODERATE | SEVERE

One Minute MIGRAINE Diary

Date : ______________________

Start Time : ________________ End Time : ____________ Duration : ________

PAIN SCALE [1-10]

1 2 3 4 5 6 7 8 9 10

MILD MODERATE SEVERE

MENSTRUAL PERIOD

YES NO

Birth Control Pills

YES NO

PAIN TYPE

Stabbing Burning Pulsating Shocking Pressure Pounding

SLEEP

WATER

MISSED MEALS

YES NO

PAIN LOCATION

FRONT BACK LEFT RIGHT TOP

WEATHER

TEMP °

STRESS

YES NO

LIGHTS

YES NO

SOUNDS

YES NO

SMELLS

YES NO

FOODS CONSUMED (within last 24 hours)

- ☐ Alcohol
- ☐ Artificial Sweetener
- ☐ Beans
- ☐ Caffeine
- ☐ Cheese
- ☐ Chocolate
- ☐ Fermented Foods
- ☐ MSG
- ☐ Non Friendly Fruits
- ☐ Nuts
- ☐ Processed Meats
- ☐
- ☐
- ☐

PRODROME (1-2 hours before headache)

- ☐ Excessive Thirst
- ☐ Excessive Yawning
- ☐ Face Sensitivity
- ☐ Irritability
- ☐ Light Sensitivity
- ☐ Neck Tightness
- ☐ Unexplained Fatigue
- ☐ Visual Disturbances
- ☐
- ☐
- ☐
- ☐
- ☐

SYMPTOMS

- ☐ Distorted Vision
- ☐ Dizziness
- ☐ Irritability
- ☐ Light-headedness
- ☐ Light Sensitivity
- ☐ Malaise
- ☐ Nasal Congestion
- ☐ Nausea/Vomiting
- ☐ Sound Sensitivity
- ☐ Tender Scalp
- ☐
- ☐
- ☐

AURA (20-30 mins before)

- ☐ Black Spots
- ☐ Flashing Lights
- ☐ Lack of Vision
- ☐ Numbness FACE ARM LEG
- ☐ Zig Zag Lines
- ☐
- ☐

TRIGGER & SYMPTOM NOTES

REMEDIES

(NATURAL)

- ☐ Acupuncture
- ☐ Acupressure
- ☐ Caffeine
- ☐ Dark Room
- ☐ Hot Compress
- ☐ Hydration
- ☐
- ☐
- ☐
- ☐ Ice Pack
- ☐ Massage
- ☐ Relaxation
- ☐ Silence
- ☐ Walk
- ☐
- ☐
- ☐
- ☐

(OTC- COUNTER MEDS)

- ☐ Excedrin
- ☐ Ibuprofen
- ☐ Tylenol
- ☐
- ☐
- ☐
- ☐
- ☐
- ☐

(Rx - PREVENTIVE)

- ☐ Amitriptyline
- ☐ Atenolol
- ☐ Gabapentin
- ☐ Nurtriptyline
- ☐ Propranolol
- ☐ Topamax
- ☐ Valproate
- ☐
- ☐

(Rx - RELIEF)

- ☐ Naproxin
- ☐ Nurtec
- ☐ Sumatriptan
- ☐ Rizatriptan
- ☐ Ubrelvy
- ☐
- ☐

(SUPPLEMENTS)

- ☐ B2
- ☐ Butterbur
- ☐ Feverfew
- ☐ Magnesium
- ☐
- ☐
- ☐

WITHIN 1 HR OF PAIN YES NO

PAIN RELIEF YES NO

REMEDY NOTES

IMPACT ON DAILY ACTIVITIES

NONE | MILD | MODERATE | SEVERE

WWW.ONEMINUTEMIGRAINEDIARY.COM

One Minute MIGRAINE Diary

Date : ____________________

Start Time : ____________ End Time : ____________ Duration : ________

PAIN SCALE [1-10]	MENSTRUAL PERIOD	PAIN TYPE	WATER
1 2 3 4 5 6 7 8 9 10 MILD MODERATE SEVERE	YES NO Birth Control Pills YES NO	Stabbing Burning Pulsating Shocking Pressure Pounding SLEEP	MISSED MEALS YES NO

PAIN LOCATION

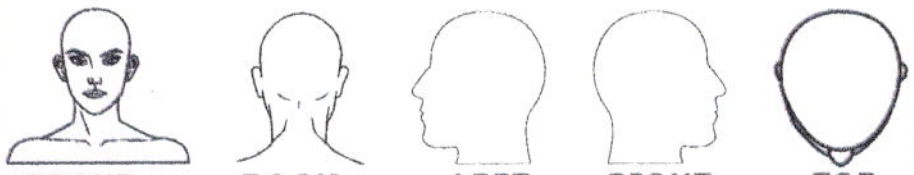

WEATHER

TEMP °

STRESS YES NO

LIGHTS YES NO **SOUNDS** YES NO

SMELLS YES NO

FOODS CONSUMED
(within last 24 hours)

- ☐ Alcohol
- ☐ Artificial Sweetener
- ☐ Beans
- ☐ Caffeine
- ☐ Cheese
- ☐ Chocolate
- ☐ Fermented Foods
- ☐ MSG
- ☐ Non Friendly Fruits
- ☐ Nuts
- ☐ Processed Meats
- ☐
- ☐
- ☐

PRODROME
(1-2 hours before headache)

- ☐ Excessive Thirst
- ☐ Excessive Yawning
- ☐ Face Sensitivity
- ☐ Irritability
- ☐ Light Sensitivity
- ☐ Neck Tightness
- ☐ Unexplained Fatigue
- ☐ Visual Disturbances
- ☐
- ☐
- ☐
- ☐
- ☐

SYMPTOMS

- ☐ Distorted Vision
- ☐ Dizziness
- ☐ Irritability
- ☐ Light-headedness
- ☐ Light Sensitivity
- ☐ Malaise
- ☐ Nasal Congestion
- ☐ Nausea/Vomiting
- ☐ Sound Sensitivity
- ☐ Tender Scalp
- ☐
- ☐
- ☐

AURA
(20-30 mins before)

- ☐ Black Spots
- ☐ Flashing Lights
- ☐ Lack of Vision
- ☐ Numbness FACE ARM LEG
- ☐ Zig Zag Lines
- ☐
- ☐

TRIGGER & SYMPTOM NOTES

REMEDIES

(NATURAL)

- ☐ Acupuncture
- ☐ Acupressure
- ☐ Caffeine
- ☐ Dark Room
- ☐ Hot Compress
- ☐ Hydration
- ☐
- ☐
- ☐
- ☐ Ice Pack
- ☐ Massage
- ☐ Relaxation
- ☐ Silence
- ☐ Walk
- ☐
- ☐
- ☐
- ☐

(OTC- COUNTER MEDS)

- ☐ Excedrin
- ☐ Ibuprofen
- ☐ Tylenol
- ☐
- ☐
- ☐
- ☐
- ☐
- ☐

(Rx - PREVENTIVE)

- ☐ Amitriptyline
- ☐ Atenolol
- ☐ Gabapentin
- ☐ Nurtriptyline
- ☐ Propranolol
- ☐ Topamax
- ☐ Valproate
- ☐
- ☐

(Rx - RELIEF)

- ☐ Naproxin
- ☐ Nurtec
- ☐ Sumatriptan
- ☐ Rizatriptan
- ☐ Ubrelvy
- ☐
- ☐

(SUPPLEMENTS)

- ☐ B2
- ☐ Butterbur
- ☐ Feverfew
- ☐ Magnesium
- ☐
- ☐
- ☐

WITHIN 1 HR OF PAIN YES NO PAIN RELIEF YES NO

REMEDY NOTES

IMPACT ON DAILY ACTIVITIES

NONE | MILD | MODERATE | SEVERE

WWW.ONEMINUTEMIGRAINEDIARY.COM

One Minute MIGRAINE Diary

Date : ____________________

Start Time : ______________ End Time : ______________ Duration : ________

PAIN SCALE [1-10]
1 2 3 4 5 6 7 8 9 10
MILD MODERATE SEVERE

MENSTRUAL PERIOD
YES NO
Birth Control Pills
YES NO

PAIN TYPE
Stabbing Burning Pulsating Shocking Pressure Pounding

SLEEP

WATER

MISSED MEALS
YES NO

PAIN LOCATION
FRONT BACK LEFT RIGHT TOP

WEATHER
° TEMP

STRESS
YES NO

LIGHTS
YES NO

SOUNDS
YES NO

SMELLS
YES NO

FOODS CONSUMED (within last 24 hours)
- ☐ Alcohol
- ☐ Artificial Sweetener
- ☐ Beans
- ☐ Caffeine
- ☐ Cheese
- ☐ Chocolate
- ☐ Fermented Foods
- ☐ MSG
- ☐ Non Friendly Fruits
- ☐ Nuts
- ☐ Processed Meats
- ☐
- ☐
- ☐

PRODROME (1-2 hours before headache)
- ☐ Excessive Thirst
- ☐ Excessive Yawning
- ☐ Face Sensitivity
- ☐ Irritability
- ☐ Light Sensitivity
- ☐ Neck Tightness
- ☐ Unexplained Fatigue
- ☐ Visual Disturbances
- ☐
- ☐
- ☐
- ☐
- ☐

SYMPTOMS
- ☐ Distorted Vision
- ☐ Dizziness
- ☐ Irritability
- ☐ Light-headedness
- ☐ Light Sensitivity
- ☐ Malaise
- ☐ Nasal Congestion
- ☐ Nausea/Vomiting
- ☐ Sound Sensitivity
- ☐ Tender Scalp
- ☐
- ☐
- ☐

AURA (20-30 mins before)
- ☐ Black Spots
- ☐ Flashing Lights
- ☐ Lack of Vision
- ☐ Numbness FACE ARM LEG
- ☐ Zig Zag Lines
- ☐
- ☐

TRIGGER & SYMPTOM NOTES

REMEDIES

(NATURAL)
- ☐ Acupuncture
- ☐ Acupressure
- ☐ Caffeine
- ☐ Dark Room
- ☐ Hot Compress
- ☐ Hydration
- ☐
- ☐
- ☐
- ☐ Ice Pack
- ☐ Massage
- ☐ Relaxation
- ☐ Silence
- ☐ Walk
- ☐
- ☐
- ☐
- ☐

(OTC- COUNTER MEDS)
- ☐ Excedrin
- ☐ Ibuprofen
- ☐ Tylenol
- ☐
- ☐
- ☐
- ☐
- ☐
- ☐

(Rx - PREVENTIVE)
- ☐ Amitriptyline
- ☐ Atenolol
- ☐ Gabapentin
- ☐ Nurtriptyline
- ☐ Propranolol
- ☐ Topamax
- ☐ Valproate
- ☐
- ☐

(Rx - RELIEF)
- ☐ Naproxin
- ☐ Nurtec
- ☐ Sumatriptan
- ☐ Rizatriptan
- ☐ Ubrelvy
- ☐
- ☐

(SUPPLEMENTS)
- ☐ B2
- ☐ Butterbur
- ☐ Feverfew
- ☐ Magnesium
- ☐
- ☐
- ☐

WITHIN 1 HR OF PAIN YES NO PAIN RELIEF YES NO

REMEDY NOTES

IMPACT ON DAILY ACTIVITIES
NONE | MILD | MODERATE | SEVERE

WWW.ONEMINUTEMIGRAINEDIARY.COM

One Minute MIGRAINE Diary

Date : ______________________

Start Time : ______________ End Time : ______________ Duration : ________

PAIN SCALE [1-10]	MENSTRUAL PERIOD	PAIN TYPE	WATER
1 2 3 4 5 6 7 8 9 10 MILD MODERATE SEVERE	YES NO Birth Control Pills YES NO	Stabbing Burning Pulsating Shocking Pressure Pounding SLEEP	MISSED MEALS YES NO

PAIN LOCATION	WEATHER	STRESS
FRONT BACK LEFT RIGHT TOP	TEMP °	YES NO
	LIGHTS YES NO / SOUNDS YES NO	SMELLS YES NO

FOODS CONSUMED (within last 24 hours)	PRODROME (1-2 hours before headache)	SYMPTOMS	AURA (20-30 mins before)
☐ Alcohol	☐ Excessive Thirst	☐ Distorted Vision	☐ Black Spots
☐ Artificial Sweetener	☐ Excessive Yawning	☐ Dizziness	☐ Flashing Lights
☐ Beans	☐ Face Sensitivity	☐ Irritability	☐ Lack of Vision
☐ Caffeine	☐ Irritability	☐ Light-headedness	☐ Numbness FACE ARM LEG
☐ Cheese	☐ Light Sensitivity	☐ Light Sensitivity	☐ Zig Zag Lines
☐ Chocolate	☐ Neck Tightness	☐ Malaise	☐
☐ Fermented Foods	☐ Unexplained Fatigue	☐ Nasal Congestion	☐
☐ MSG	☐ Visual Disturbances	☐ Nausea/Vomiting	TRIGGER & SYMPTOM NOTES
☐ Non Friendly Fruits	☐	☐ Sound Sensitivity	
☐ Nuts	☐	☐ Tender Scalp	
☐ Processed Meats	☐	☐	
☐	☐	☐	
☐	☐	☐	
☐	☐		

REMEDIES

(NATURAL)		(OTC- COUNTER MEDS)	(Rx - PREVENTIVE)	(Rx - RELIEF)	(SUPPLEMENTS)
☐ Acupuncture	☐ Ice Pack	☐ Excedrin	☐ Amitriptyline	☐ Naproxin	☐ B2
☐ Acupressure	☐ Massage	☐ Ibuprofen	☐ Atenolol	☐ Nurtec	☐ Butterbur
☐ Caffeine	☐ Relaxation	☐ Tylenol	☐ Gabapentin	☐ Sumatriptan	☐ Feverfew
☐ Dark Room	☐ Silence	☐	☐ Nurtriptyline	☐ Rizatriptan	☐ Magnesium
☐ Hot Compress	☐ Walk	☐	☐ Propranolol	☐ Ubrelvy	☐
☐ Hydration	☐	☐	☐ Topamax	☐	☐
☐	☐	☐	☐ Valproate	☐	☐
☐	☐	☐	☐	WITHIN 1 HR OF PAIN YES NO	PAIN RELIEF YES NO
☐	☐	☐	☐		

REMEDY NOTES

IMPACT ON DAILY ACTIVITIES

NONE | MILD | MODERATE | SEVERE

WWW.ONEMINUTEMIGRAINEDIARY.COM

One Minute MIGRAINE Diary

Date : ____________________

Start Time : ______________ End Time : ______________ Duration : ______

PAIN SCALE [1-10]
1 2 3 4 5 6 7 8 9 10
MILD MODERATE SEVERE

MENSTRUAL PERIOD
YES NO
Birth Control Pills
YES NO

PAIN TYPE
Stabbing Burning Pulsating Shocking Pressure Pounding

SLEEP

WATER

MISSED MEALS
YES NO

PAIN LOCATION
FRONT BACK LEFT RIGHT TOP

WEATHER
TEMP °

STRESS
YES NO

LIGHTS
YES NO

SOUNDS
YES NO

SMELLS
YES NO

FOODS CONSUMED (within last 24 hours)
- ☐ Alcohol
- ☐ Artificial Sweetener
- ☐ Beans
- ☐ Caffeine
- ☐ Cheese
- ☐ Chocolate
- ☐ Fermented Foods
- ☐ MSG
- ☐ Non Friendly Fruits
- ☐ Nuts
- ☐ Processed Meats
- ☐
- ☐
- ☐

PRODROME (1-2 hours before headache)
- ☐ Excessive Thirst
- ☐ Excessive Yawning
- ☐ Face Sensitivity
- ☐ Irritability
- ☐ Light Sensitivity
- ☐ Neck Tightness
- ☐ Unexplained Fatigue
- ☐ Visual Disturbances
- ☐
- ☐
- ☐
- ☐
- ☐

SYMPTOMS
- ☐ Distorted Vision
- ☐ Dizziness
- ☐ Irritability
- ☐ Light-headedness
- ☐ Light Sensitivity
- ☐ Malaise
- ☐ Nasal Congestion
- ☐ Nausea/Vomiting
- ☐ Sound Sensitivity
- ☐ Tender Scalp
- ☐
- ☐
- ☐

AURA (20-30 mins before)
- ☐ Black Spots
- ☐ Flashing Lights
- ☐ Lack of Vision
- ☐ Numbness FACE ARM LEG
- ☐ Zig Zag Lines
- ☐
- ☐

TRIGGER & SYMPTOM NOTES

REMEDIES

(NATURAL)
- ☐ Acupuncture
- ☐ Acupressure
- ☐ Caffeine
- ☐ Dark Room
- ☐ Hot Compress
- ☐ Hydration
- ☐
- ☐
- ☐
- ☐ Ice Pack
- ☐ Massage
- ☐ Relaxation
- ☐ Silence
- ☐ Walk
- ☐
- ☐
- ☐
- ☐

(OTC- COUNTER MEDS)
- ☐ Excedrin
- ☐ Ibuprofen
- ☐ Tylenol
- ☐
- ☐
- ☐
- ☐
- ☐
- ☐

(Rx - PREVENTIVE)
- ☐ Amitriptyline
- ☐ Atenolol
- ☐ Gabapentin
- ☐ Nurtriptyline
- ☐ Propranolol
- ☐ Topamax
- ☐ Valproate
- ☐
- ☐

(Rx - RELIEF)
- ☐ Naproxin
- ☐ Nurtec
- ☐ Sumatriptan
- ☐ Rizatriptan
- ☐ Ubrelvy
- ☐
- ☐

(SUPPLEMENTS)
- ☐ B2
- ☐ Butterbur
- ☐ Feverfew
- ☐ Magnesium
- ☐
- ☐
- ☐

WITHIN 1 HR OF PAIN YES NO PAIN RELIEF YES NO

REMEDY NOTES

IMPACT ON DAILY ACTIVITIES
NONE | MILD | MODERATE | SEVERE

WWW.ONEMINUTEMIGRAINEDIARY.COM

One Minute MIGRAINE Diary

Date : ____________________

Start Time : ______________ End Time : ____________ Duration : ______

PAIN SCALE [1-10]	MENSTRUAL PERIOD	PAIN TYPE	WATER
1 2 3 4 5 6 7 8 9 10 MILD MODERATE SEVERE	YES NO Birth Control Pills YES NO	Stabbing Burning Pulsating Shocking Pressure Pounding SLEEP	MISSED MEALS YES NO

PAIN LOCATION	WEATHER	STRESS
FRONT BACK LEFT RIGHT TOP	TEMP °	YES NO
	LIGHTS YES NO / SOUNDS YES NO	SMELLS YES NO

FOODS CONSUMED (within last 24 hours)	PRODROME (1-2 hours before headache)	SYMPTOMS	AURA (20-30 mins before)
☐ Alcohol	☐ Excessive Thirst	☐ Distorted Vision	☐ Black Spots
☐ Artificial Sweetener	☐ Excessive Yawning	☐ Dizziness	☐ Flashing Lights
☐ Beans	☐ Face Sensitivity	☐ Irritability	☐ Lack of Vision
☐ Caffeine	☐ Irritability	☐ Light-headedness	☐ Numbness FACE ARM LEG
☐ Cheese	☐ Light Sensitivity	☐ Light Sensitivity	☐ Zig Zag Lines
☐ Chocolate	☐ Neck Tightness	☐ Malaise	☐
☐ Fermented Foods	☐ Unexplained Fatigue	☐ Nasal Congestion	☐
☐ MSG	☐ Visual Disturbances	☐ Nausea/Vomiting	TRIGGER & SYMPTOM NOTES
☐ Non Friendly Fruits	☐	☐ Sound Sensitivity	
☐ Nuts	☐	☐ Tender Scalp	
☐ Processed Meats	☐	☐	
☐	☐	☐	
☐	☐	☐	
☐			

REMEDIES

(NATURAL)		(OTC- COUNTER MEDS)	(Rx - PREVENTIVE)	(Rx - RELIEF)	(SUPPLEMENTS)
☐ Acupuncture	☐ Ice Pack	☐ Excedrin	☐ Amitriptyline	☐ Naproxin	☐ B2
☐ Acupressure	☐ Massage	☐ Ibuprofen	☐ Atenolol	☐ Nurtec	☐ Butterbur
☐ Caffeine	☐ Relaxation	☐ Tylenol	☐ Gabapentin	☐ Sumatriptan	☐ Feverfew
☐ Dark Room	☐ Silence	☐	☐ Nurtriptyline	☐ Rizatriptan	☐ Magnesium
☐ Hot Compress	☐ Walk	☐	☐ Propranolol	☐ Ubrelvy	☐
☐ Hydration	☐	☐	☐ Topamax	☐	☐
☐	☐	☐	☐ Valproate	☐	☐
☐	☐	☐	☐	WITHIN 1 HR OF PAIN YES NO	PAIN RELIEF YES NO
☐	☐	☐	☐		

REMEDY NOTES

IMPACT ON DAILY ACTIVITIES

NONE | MILD | MODERATE | SEVERE

WWW.ONEMINUTEMIGRAINEDIARY.COM

One Minute MIGRAINE Diary

Date : ____________________

Start Time : ______________ End Time : ____________ Duration : ________

PAIN SCALE [1-10]

1 2 3 4 5 6 7 8 9 10

MILD MODERATE SEVERE

MENSTRUAL PERIOD

YES NO

Birth Control Pills

YES NO

PAIN TYPE

Stabbing Burning Pulsating Shocking Pressure Pounding

SLEEP

WATER

MISSED MEALS

YES NO

PAIN LOCATION

FRONT BACK LEFT RIGHT TOP

WEATHER

TEMP °

STRESS

YES NO

LIGHTS

YES NO

SOUNDS

YES NO

SMELLS

YES NO

FOODS CONSUMED (within last 24 hours)

- ☐ Alcohol
- ☐ Artificial Sweetener
- ☐ Beans
- ☐ Caffeine
- ☐ Cheese
- ☐ Chocolate
- ☐ Fermented Foods
- ☐ MSG
- ☐ Non Friendly Fruits
- ☐ Nuts
- ☐ Processed Meats
- ☐
- ☐
- ☐

PRODROME (1-2 hours before headache)

- ☐ Excessive Thirst
- ☐ Excessive Yawning
- ☐ Face Sensitivity
- ☐ Irritability
- ☐ Light Sensitivity
- ☐ Neck Tightness
- ☐ Unexplained Fatigue
- ☐ Visual Disturbances
- ☐
- ☐
- ☐
- ☐
- ☐

SYMPTOMS

- ☐ Distorted Vision
- ☐ Dizziness
- ☐ Irritability
- ☐ Light-headedness
- ☐ Light Sensitivity
- ☐ Malaise
- ☐ Nasal Congestion
- ☐ Nausea/Vomiting
- ☐ Sound Sensitivity
- ☐ Tender Scalp
- ☐
- ☐
- ☐

AURA (20-30 mins before)

- ☐ Black Spots
- ☐ Flashing Lights
- ☐ Lack of Vision
- ☐ Numbness FACE ARM LEG
- ☐ Zig Zag Lines
- ☐
- ☐

TRIGGER & SYMPTOM NOTES

REMEDIES

(NATURAL)

- ☐ Acupuncture
- ☐ Acupressure
- ☐ Caffeine
- ☐ Dark Room
- ☐ Hot Compress
- ☐ Hydration
- ☐
- ☐
- ☐
- ☐ Ice Pack
- ☐ Massage
- ☐ Relaxation
- ☐ Silence
- ☐ Walk
- ☐
- ☐
- ☐
- ☐

(OTC- COUNTER MEDS)

- ☐ Excedrin
- ☐ Ibuprofen
- ☐ Tylenol
- ☐
- ☐
- ☐
- ☐
- ☐
- ☐

(Rx - PREVENTIVE)

- ☐ Amitriptyline
- ☐ Atenolol
- ☐ Gabapentin
- ☐ Nurtriptyline
- ☐ Propranolol
- ☐ Topamax
- ☐ Valproate
- ☐
- ☐

(Rx - RELIEF)

- ☐ Naproxin
- ☐ Nurtec
- ☐ Sumatriptan
- ☐ Rizatriptan
- ☐ Ubrelvy
- ☐
- ☐

(SUPPLEMENTS)

- ☐ B2
- ☐ Butterbur
- ☐ Feverfew
- ☐ Magnesium
- ☐
- ☐
- ☐

WITHIN 1 HR OF PAIN YES NO

PAIN RELIEF YES NO

REMEDY NOTES

IMPACT ON DAILY ACTIVITIES

NONE | MILD | MODERATE | SEVERE

WWW.ONEMINUTEMIGRAINEDIARY.COM

One Minute MIGRAINE Diary

Date : ____________________

Start Time : ____________ End Time : ____________ Duration : ________

PAIN SCALE [1-10]	MENSTRUAL PERIOD	PAIN TYPE	WATER
1 2 3 4 5 6 7 8 9 10 MILD MODERATE SEVERE	YES NO Birth Control Pills YES NO	Stabbing Burning Pulsating Shocking Pressure Pounding SLEEP	MISSED MEALS YES NO

PAIN LOCATION	WEATHER	STRESS
FRONT BACK LEFT RIGHT TOP	TEMP °	YES NO
	LIGHTS YES NO / SOUNDS YES NO	SMELLS YES NO

FOODS CONSUMED (within last 24 hours)	PRODROME (1-2 hours before headache)	SYMPTOMS	AURA (20-30 mins before)
☐ Alcohol	☐ Excessive Thirst	☐ Distorted Vision	☐ Black Spots
☐ Artificial Sweetener	☐ Excessive Yawning	☐ Dizziness	☐ Flashing Lights
☐ Beans	☐ Face Sensitivity	☐ Irritability	☐ Lack of Vision
☐ Caffeine	☐ Irritability	☐ Light-headedness	☐ Numbness FACE ARM LEG
☐ Cheese	☐ Light Sensitivity	☐ Light Sensitivity	☐ Zig Zag Lines
☐ Chocolate	☐ Neck Tightness	☐ Malaise	☐
☐ Fermented Foods	☐ Unexplained Fatigue	☐ Nasal Congestion	☐
☐ MSG	☐ Visual Disturbances	☐ Nausea/Vomiting	TRIGGER & SYMPTOM NOTES
☐ Non Friendly Fruits	☐	☐ Sound Sensitivity	
☐ Nuts	☐	☐ Tender Scalp	
☐ Processed Meats	☐	☐	
☐	☐	☐	
☐	☐	☐	
☐	☐		

REMEDIES

(NATURAL)		(OTC- COUNTER MEDS)	(Rx - PREVENTIVE)	(Rx - RELIEF)	(SUPPLEMENTS)
☐ Acupuncture	☐ Ice Pack	☐ Excedrin	☐ Amitriptyline	☐ Naproxin	☐ B2
☐ Acupressure	☐ Massage	☐ Ibuprofen	☐ Atenolol	☐ Nurtec	☐ Butterbur
☐ Caffeine	☐ Relaxation	☐ Tylenol	☐ Gabapentin	☐ Sumatriptan	☐ Feverfew
☐ Dark Room	☐ Silence	☐	☐ Nurtriptyline	☐ Rizatriptan	☐ Magnesium
☐ Hot Compress	☐ Walk	☐	☐ Propranolol	☐ Ubrelvy	☐
☐ Hydration	☐	☐	☐ Topamax	☐	☐
☐	☐	☐	☐ Valproate	☐	☐
☐	☐	☐	☐	WITHIN 1 HR OF PAIN YES NO	PAIN RELIEF YES NO
☐	☐	☐	☐		

REMEDY NOTES

IMPACT ON DAILY ACTIVITIES

NONE | MILD | MODERATE | SEVERE

WWW.ONEMINUTEMIGRAINEDIARY.COM

One Minute MIGRAINE Diary

Date : ____________________

Start Time : ______________ End Time : ______________ Duration : ________

PAIN SCALE [1-10]

|-----|-----|-----|-----|-----|-----|-----|-----|-----|
1 2 3 4 5 6 7 8 9 10
MILD MODERATE SEVERE

MENSTRUAL PERIOD
YES NO
Birth Control Pills
YES NO

PAIN TYPE
Stabbing Burning Pulsating Shocking Pressure Pounding

SLEEP

WATER

MISSED MEALS
YES NO

PAIN LOCATION
FRONT BACK LEFT RIGHT TOP

WEATHER
TEMP °

STRESS
YES NO

LIGHTS
YES NO

SOUNDS
YES NO

SMELLS
YES NO

FOODS CONSUMED (within last 24 hours)
- ☐ Alcohol
- ☐ Artificial Sweetener
- ☐ Beans
- ☐ Caffeine
- ☐ Cheese
- ☐ Chocolate
- ☐ Fermented Foods
- ☐ MSG
- ☐ Non Friendly Fruits
- ☐ Nuts
- ☐ Processed Meats
- ☐
- ☐
- ☐

PRODROME (1-2 hours before headache)
- ☐ Excessive Thirst
- ☐ Excessive Yawning
- ☐ Face Sensitivity
- ☐ Irritability
- ☐ Light Sensitivity
- ☐ Neck Tightness
- ☐ Unexplained Fatigue
- ☐ Visual Disturbances
- ☐
- ☐
- ☐
- ☐
- ☐

SYMPTOMS
- ☐ Distorted Vision
- ☐ Dizziness
- ☐ Irritability
- ☐ Light-headedness
- ☐ Light Sensitivity
- ☐ Malaise
- ☐ Nasal Congestion
- ☐ Nausea/Vomiting
- ☐ Sound Sensitivity
- ☐ Tender Scalp
- ☐
- ☐
- ☐

AURA (20-30 mins before)
- ☐ Black Spots
- ☐ Flashing Lights
- ☐ Lack of Vision
- ☐ Numbness FACE ARM LEG
- ☐ Zig Zag Lines
- ☐
- ☐

TRIGGER & SYMPTOM NOTES

REMEDIES

(NATURAL)
- ☐ Acupuncture
- ☐ Acupressure
- ☐ Caffeine
- ☐ Dark Room
- ☐ Hot Compress
- ☐ Hydration
- ☐
- ☐
- ☐
- ☐ Ice Pack
- ☐ Massage
- ☐ Relaxation
- ☐ Silence
- ☐ Walk
- ☐
- ☐
- ☐
- ☐

(OTC- COUNTER MEDS)
- ☐ Excedrin
- ☐ Ibuprofen
- ☐ Tylenol
- ☐
- ☐
- ☐
- ☐
- ☐
- ☐

(Rx - PREVENTIVE)
- ☐ Amitriptyline
- ☐ Atenolol
- ☐ Gabapentin
- ☐ Nurtriptyline
- ☐ Propranolol
- ☐ Topamax
- ☐ Valproate
- ☐
- ☐

(Rx - RELIEF)
- ☐ Naproxin
- ☐ Nurtec
- ☐ Sumatriptan
- ☐ Rizatriptan
- ☐ Ubrelvy
- ☐
- ☐

(SUPPLEMENTS)
- ☐ B2
- ☐ Butterbur
- ☐ Feverfew
- ☐ Magnesium
- ☐
- ☐
- ☐

WITHIN 1 HR OF PAIN YES NO PAIN RELIEF YES NO

REMEDY NOTES

IMPACT ON DAILY ACTIVITIES
NONE | MILD | MODERATE | SEVERE

WWW.ONEMINUTEMIGRAINEDIARY.COM

One Minute MIGRAINE Diary

Date : ______________________________

Start Time : ________________ End Time : ________________ Duration : ________

PAIN SCALE [1-10]

|-----|-----|-----|-----|-----|-----|-----|-----|-----|
1 2 3 4 5 6 7 8 9 10
MILD MODERATE SEVERE

MENSTRUAL PERIOD

YES NO

Birth Control Pills

YES NO

PAIN TYPE

Stabbing Burning Pulsating Shocking Pressure Pounding

SLEEP

WATER

MISSED MEALS

YES NO

PAIN LOCATION

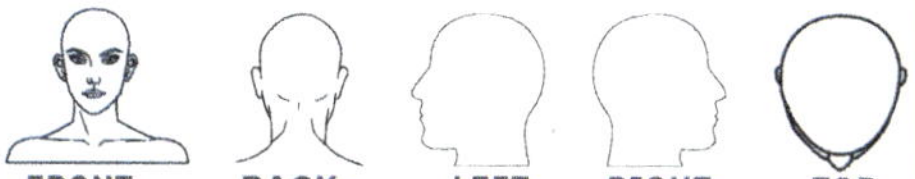

FRONT BACK LEFT RIGHT TOP

WEATHER

TEMP °

STRESS

YES NO

LIGHTS

YES NO

SOUNDS

YES NO

SMELLS

YES NO

FOODS CONSUMED (within last 24 hours)

- ☐ Alcohol
- ☐ Artificial Sweetener
- ☐ Beans
- ☐ Caffeine
- ☐ Cheese
- ☐ Chocolate
- ☐ Fermented Foods
- ☐ MSG
- ☐ Non Friendly Fruits
- ☐ Nuts
- ☐ Processed Meats
- ☐
- ☐
- ☐

PRODROME (1-2 hours before headache)

- ☐ Excessive Thirst
- ☐ Excessive Yawning
- ☐ Face Sensitivity
- ☐ Irritability
- ☐ Light Sensitivity
- ☐ Neck Tightness
- ☐ Unexplained Fatigue
- ☐ Visual Disturbances
- ☐
- ☐
- ☐
- ☐
- ☐

SYMPTOMS

- ☐ Distorted Vision
- ☐ Dizziness
- ☐ Irritability
- ☐ Light-headedness
- ☐ Light Sensitivity
- ☐ Malaise
- ☐ Nasal Congestion
- ☐ Nausea/Vomiting
- ☐ Sound Sensitivity
- ☐ Tender Scalp
- ☐
- ☐
- ☐

AURA (20-30 mins before)

- ☐ Black Spots
- ☐ Flashing Lights
- ☐ Lack of Vision
- ☐ Numbness FACE ARM LEG
- ☐ Zig Zag Lines
- ☐
- ☐

TRIGGER & SYMPTOM NOTES

REMEDIES

(NATURAL)

- ☐ Acupuncture
- ☐ Acupressure
- ☐ Caffeine
- ☐ Dark Room
- ☐ Hot Compress
- ☐ Hydration
- ☐
- ☐
- ☐
- ☐ Ice Pack
- ☐ Massage
- ☐ Relaxation
- ☐ Silence
- ☐ Walk
- ☐
- ☐
- ☐
- ☐

(OTC- COUNTER MEDS)

- ☐ Excedrin
- ☐ Ibuprofen
- ☐ Tylenol
- ☐
- ☐
- ☐
- ☐
- ☐
- ☐

(Rx - PREVENTIVE)

- ☐ Amitriptyline
- ☐ Atenolol
- ☐ Gabapentin
- ☐ Nurtriptyline
- ☐ Propranolol
- ☐ Topamax
- ☐ Valproate
- ☐
- ☐

(Rx - RELIEF)

- ☐ Naproxin
- ☐ Nurtec
- ☐ Sumatriptan
- ☐ Rizatriptan
- ☐ Ubrelvy
- ☐
- ☐

(SUPPLEMENTS)

- ☐ B2
- ☐ Butterbur
- ☐ Feverfew
- ☐ Magnesium
- ☐
- ☐
- ☐

WITHIN 1 HR OF PAIN YES NO

PAIN RELIEF YES NO

REMEDY NOTES

IMPACT ON DAILY ACTIVITIES

NONE | MILD | MODERATE | SEVERE

WWW.ONEMINUTEMIGRAINEDIARY.COM

One Minute MIGRAINE Diary

Date : ______________________

Start Time : ______________ End Time : ______________ Duration : __________

PAIN SCALE [1-10]

1 2 3 4 5 6 7 8 9 10
MILD MODERATE SEVERE

MENSTRUAL PERIOD
YES NO
Birth Control Pills
YES NO

PAIN TYPE
Stabbing Burning Pulsating Shocking Pressure Pounding

SLEEP

WATER

MISSED MEALS
YES NO

PAIN LOCATION
FRONT BACK LEFT RIGHT TOP

WEATHER
° TEMP

STRESS
YES NO

LIGHTS
YES NO

SOUNDS
YES NO

SMELLS
YES NO

FOODS CONSUMED (within last 24 hours)
- ☐ Alcohol
- ☐ Artificial Sweetener
- ☐ Beans
- ☐ Caffeine
- ☐ Cheese
- ☐ Chocolate
- ☐ Fermented Foods
- ☐ MSG
- ☐ Non Friendly Fruits
- ☐ Nuts
- ☐ Processed Meats
- ☐
- ☐
- ☐

PRODROME (1-2 hours before headache)
- ☐ Excessive Thirst
- ☐ Excessive Yawning
- ☐ Face Sensitivity
- ☐ Irritability
- ☐ Light Sensitivity
- ☐ Neck Tightness
- ☐ Unexplained Fatigue
- ☐ Visual Disturbances
- ☐
- ☐
- ☐
- ☐
- ☐

SYMPTOMS
- ☐ Distorted Vision
- ☐ Dizziness
- ☐ Irritability
- ☐ Light-headedness
- ☐ Light Sensitivity
- ☐ Malaise
- ☐ Nasal Congestion
- ☐ Nausea/Vomiting
- ☐ Sound Sensitivity
- ☐ Tender Scalp
- ☐
- ☐
- ☐

AURA (20-30 mins before)
- ☐ Black Spots
- ☐ Flashing Lights
- ☐ Lack of Vision
- ☐ Numbness FACE ARM LEG
- ☐ Zig Zag Lines
- ☐
- ☐

TRIGGER & SYMPTOM NOTES

REMEDIES

(NATURAL)
- ☐ Acupuncture
- ☐ Acupressure
- ☐ Caffeine
- ☐ Dark Room
- ☐ Hot Compress
- ☐ Hydration
- ☐
- ☐
- ☐
- ☐ Ice Pack
- ☐ Massage
- ☐ Relaxation
- ☐ Silence
- ☐ Walk
- ☐
- ☐
- ☐
- ☐

(OTC- COUNTER MEDS)
- ☐ Excedrin
- ☐ Ibuprofen
- ☐ Tylenol
- ☐
- ☐
- ☐
- ☐
- ☐
- ☐

(Rx - PREVENTIVE)
- ☐ Amitriptyline
- ☐ Atenolol
- ☐ Gabapentin
- ☐ Nurtriptyline
- ☐ Propranolol
- ☐ Topamax
- ☐ Valproate
- ☐
- ☐

(Rx - RELIEF)
- ☐ Naproxin
- ☐ Nurtec
- ☐ Sumatriptan
- ☐ Rizatriptan
- ☐ Ubrelvy
- ☐
- ☐

(SUPPLEMENTS)
- ☐ B2
- ☐ Butterbur
- ☐ Feverfew
- ☐ Magnesium
- ☐
- ☐
- ☐

WITHIN 1 HR OF PAIN YES NO PAIN RELIEF YES NO

REMEDY NOTES

IMPACT ON DAILY ACTIVITIES
NONE | MILD | MODERATE | SEVERE

WWW.ONEMINUTEMIGRAINEDIARY.COM

One Minute MIGRAINE Diary

Date : ______________________

Start Time : ______________ End Time : ______________ Duration : ________

PAIN SCALE [1-10]	MENSTRUAL PERIOD	PAIN TYPE	WATER
1 2 3 4 5 6 7 8 9 10 MILD MODERATE SEVERE	YES NO Birth Control Pills YES NO	Stabbing Burning Pulsating Shocking Pressure Pounding **SLEEP**	**MISSED MEALS** YES NO
PAIN LOCATION FRONT BACK LEFT RIGHT TOP		**WEATHER** TEMP °	**STRESS** YES NO
		LIGHTS YES NO **SOUNDS** YES NO	**SMELLS** YES NO

FOODS CONSUMED (within last 24 hours)	PRODROME (1-2 hours before headache)	SYMPTOMS	AURA (20-30 mins before)
☐ Alcohol	☐ Excessive Thirst	☐ Distorted Vision	☐ Black Spots
☐ Artificial Sweetener	☐ Excessive Yawning	☐ Dizziness	☐ Flashing Lights
☐ Beans	☐ Face Sensitivity	☐ Irritability	☐ Lack of Vision
☐ Caffeine	☐ Irritability	☐ Light-headedness	☐ Numbness FACE ARM LEG
☐ Cheese	☐ Light Sensitivity	☐ Light Sensitivity	☐ Zig Zag Lines
☐ Chocolate	☐ Neck Tightness	☐ Malaise	☐
☐ Fermented Foods	☐ Unexplained Fatigue	☐ Nasal Congestion	☐
☐ MSG	☐ Visual Disturbances	☐ Nausea/Vomiting	**TRIGGER & SYMPTOM NOTES**
☐ Non Friendly Fruits	☐	☐ Sound Sensitivity	
☐ Nuts	☐	☐ Tender Scalp	
☐ Processed Meats	☐	☐	
☐	☐	☐	
☐	☐	☐	
☐	☐		

REMEDIES

(NATURAL)		(OTC- COUNTER MEDS)	(Rx - PREVENTIVE)	(Rx - RELIEF)	(SUPPLEMENTS)
☐ Acupuncture	☐ Ice Pack	☐ Excedrin	☐ Amitriptyline	☐ Naproxin	☐ B2
☐ Acupressure	☐ Massage	☐ Ibuprofen	☐ Atenolol	☐ Nurtec	☐ Butterbur
☐ Caffeine	☐ Relaxation	☐ Tylenol	☐ Gabapentin	☐ Sumatriptan	☐ Feverfew
☐ Dark Room	☐ Silence	☐	☐ Nurtriptyline	☐ Rizatriptan	☐ Magnesium
☐ Hot Compress	☐ Walk	☐	☐ Propranolol	☐ Ubrelvy	☐
☐ Hydration	☐	☐	☐ Topamax	☐	☐
☐	☐	☐	☐ Valproate	☐	☐
☐	☐	☐	☐	WITHIN 1 HR OF PAIN YES NO	PAIN RELIEF YES NO
☐	☐	☐	☐		

REMEDY NOTES

IMPACT ON DAILY ACTIVITIES

NONE | MILD | MODERATE | SEVERE

WWW.ONEMINUTEMIGRAINEDIARY.COM

One Minute MIGRAINE Diary

Date : ____________

Start Time : ____________ End Time : ____________ Duration : ____________

PAIN SCALE [1-10]

1 2 3 4 5 6 7 8 9 10

MILD MODERATE SEVERE

MENSTRUAL PERIOD

YES NO

Birth Control Pills

YES NO

PAIN TYPE

Stabbing Burning Pulsating Shocking Pressure Pounding

SLEEP

WATER

MISSED MEALS

YES NO

PAIN LOCATION

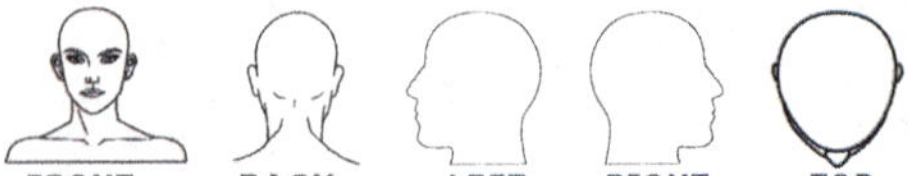

FRONT BACK LEFT RIGHT TOP

WEATHER

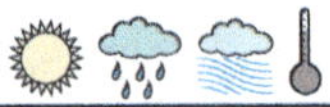

TEMP °

STRESS

YES NO

LIGHTS

YES NO

SOUNDS

YES NO

SMELLS

YES NO

FOODS CONSUMED (within last 24 hours)	PRODROME (1-2 hours before headache)	SYMPTOMS	AURA (20-30 mins before)
☐ Alcohol	☐ Excessive Thirst	☐ Distorted Vision	☐ Black Spots
☐ Artificial Sweetener	☐ Excessive Yawning	☐ Dizziness	☐ Flashing Lights
☐ Beans	☐ Face Sensitivity	☐ Irritability	☐ Lack of Vision
☐ Caffeine	☐ Irritability	☐ Light-headedness	☐ Numbness FACE ARM LEG
☐ Cheese	☐ Light Sensitivity	☐ Light Sensitivity	☐ Zig Zag Lines
☐ Chocolate	☐ Neck Tightness	☐ Malaise	☐
☐ Fermented Foods	☐ Unexplained Fatigue	☐ Nasal Congestion	☐
☐ MSG	☐ Visual Disturbances	☐ Nausea/Vomiting	TRIGGER & SYMPTOM NOTES
☐ Non Friendly Fruits	☐	☐ Sound Sensitivity	
☐ Nuts	☐	☐ Tender Scalp	
☐ Processed Meats	☐	☐	
☐	☐	☐	
☐	☐	☐	
☐	☐		

REMEDIES

(NATURAL)		(OTC- COUNTER MEDS)	(Rx - PREVENTIVE)	(Rx - RELIEF)	(SUPPLEMENTS)
☐ Acupuncture	☐ Ice Pack	☐ Excedrin	☐ Amitriptyline	☐ Naproxin	☐ B2
☐ Acupressure	☐ Massage	☐ Ibuprofen	☐ Atenolol	☐ Nurtec	☐ Butterbur
☐ Caffeine	☐ Relaxation	☐ Tylenol	☐ Gabapentin	☐ Sumatriptan	☐ Feverfew
☐ Dark Room	☐ Silence	☐	☐ Nurtriptyline	☐ Rizatriptan	☐ Magnesium
☐ Hot Compress	☐ Walk	☐	☐ Propranolol	☐ Ubrelvy	☐
☐ Hydration	☐	☐	☐ Topamax	☐	☐
☐	☐	☐	☐ Valproate	☐	☐
☐	☐	☐	☐	WITHIN 1 HR OF PAIN YES NO	PAIN RELIEF YES NO
☐	☐	☐	☐		

REMEDY NOTES

IMPACT ON DAILY ACTIVITIES

NONE | MILD | MODERATE | SEVERE

WWW.ONEMINUTEMIGRAINEDIARY.COM

One Minute MIGRAINE Diary

Date : ______________________

Start Time : ______________ End Time : ____________ Duration : ________

PAIN SCALE [1-10]	MENSTRUAL PERIOD	PAIN TYPE	WATER
1 2 3 4 5 6 7 8 9 10 MILD MODERATE SEVERE	YES NO Birth Control Pills YES NO	Stabbing Burning Pulsating Shocking Pressure Pounding SLEEP	MISSED MEALS YES NO

PAIN LOCATION	WEATHER	STRESS
FRONT BACK LEFT RIGHT TOP	° TEMP	YES NO
	LIGHTS YES NO / SOUNDS YES NO	SMELLS YES NO

FOODS CONSUMED (within last 24 hours)	PRODROME (1-2 hours before headache)	SYMPTOMS	AURA (20-30 mins before)
☐ Alcohol	☐ Excessive Thirst	☐ Distorted Vision	☐ Black Spots
☐ Artificial Sweetener	☐ Excessive Yawning	☐ Dizziness	☐ Flashing Lights
☐ Beans	☐ Face Sensitivity	☐ Irritability	☐ Lack of Vision
☐ Caffeine	☐ Irritability	☐ Light-headedness	☐ Numbness FACE ARM LEG
☐ Cheese	☐ Light Sensitivity	☐ Light Sensitivity	☐ Zig Zag Lines
☐ Chocolate	☐ Neck Tightness	☐ Malaise	☐
☐ Fermented Foods	☐ Unexplained Fatigue	☐ Nasal Congestion	☐
☐ MSG	☐ Visual Disturbances	☐ Nausea/Vomiting	TRIGGER & SYMPTOM NOTES
☐ Non Friendly Fruits	☐	☐ Sound Sensitivity	
☐ Nuts	☐	☐ Tender Scalp	
☐ Processed Meats	☐	☐	
☐	☐	☐	
☐	☐	☐	
☐	☐		

REMEDIES

(NATURAL)		(OTC- COUNTER MEDS)	(Rx - PREVENTIVE)	(Rx - RELIEF)	(SUPPLEMENTS)
☐ Acupuncture	☐ Ice Pack	☐ Excedrin	☐ Amitriptyline	☐ Naproxin	☐ B2
☐ Acupressure	☐ Massage	☐ Ibuprofen	☐ Atenolol	☐ Nurtec	☐ Butterbur
☐ Caffeine	☐ Relaxation	☐ Tylenol	☐ Gabapentin	☐ Sumatriptan	☐ Feverfew
☐ Dark Room	☐ Silence	☐	☐ Nurtriptyline	☐ Rizatriptan	☐ Magnesium
☐ Hot Compress	☐ Walk	☐	☐ Propranolol	☐ Ubrelvy	☐
☐ Hydration	☐	☐	☐ Topamax	☐	☐
☐	☐	☐	☐ Valproate	☐	☐
☐	☐	☐	☐	WITHIN 1 HR OF PAIN YES NO	PAIN RELIEF YES NO
☐	☐	☐	☐		

REMEDY NOTES

IMPACT ON DAILY ACTIVITIES

NONE | MILD | MODERATE | SEVERE

WWW.ONEMINUTEMIGRAINEDIARY.COM

One Minute MIGRAINE Diary

Month

Migraine Tracking Prompts, Reflections and Assessments To Help You Track and Manage Your Migraines

WWW.ONEMINUTEMIGRAINEDIARY.COM

I am not my pain
My pain does not define me
I am not my pain
I am not defined by my pain
I am not my pain
I am strong, capable and confident

One Minute MIGRAINE Diary

Date : ____________________

Start Time : ______________ End Time : ____________ Duration : ________

PAIN SCALE [1-10]
|-----|-----|-----|-----|-----|-----|-----|-----|-----|
1 2 3 4 5 6 7 8 9 10
MILD MODERATE SEVERE

MENSTRUAL PERIOD
YES NO
Birth Control Pills
YES NO

PAIN TYPE
Stabbing Burning Pulsating Shocking Pressure Pounding

SLEEP

WATER

MISSED MEALS
YES NO

PAIN LOCATION
FRONT BACK LEFT RIGHT TOP

WEATHER
TEMP °

STRESS
YES NO

LIGHTS
YES NO

SOUNDS
YES NO

SMELLS
YES NO

FOODS CONSUMED (within last 24 hours)
- ☐ Alcohol
- ☐ Artificial Sweetener
- ☐ Beans
- ☐ Caffeine
- ☐ Cheese
- ☐ Chocolate
- ☐ Fermented Foods
- ☐ MSG
- ☐ Non Friendly Fruits
- ☐ Nuts
- ☐ Processed Meats
- ☐
- ☐
- ☐

PRODROME (1-2 hours before headache)
- ☐ Excessive Thirst
- ☐ Excessive Yawning
- ☐ Face Sensitivity
- ☐ Irritability
- ☐ Light Sensitivity
- ☐ Neck Tightness
- ☐ Unexplained Fatigue
- ☐ Visual Disturbances
- ☐
- ☐
- ☐
- ☐
- ☐

SYMPTOMS
- ☐ Distorted Vision
- ☐ Dizziness
- ☐ Irritability
- ☐ Light-headedness
- ☐ Light Sensitivity
- ☐ Malaise
- ☐ Nasal Congestion
- ☐ Nausea/Vomiting
- ☐ Sound Sensitivity
- ☐ Tender Scalp
- ☐
- ☐
- ☐

AURA (20-30 mins before)
- ☐ Black Spots
- ☐ Flashing Lights
- ☐ Lack of Vision
- ☐ Numbness FACE ARM LEG
- ☐ Zig Zag Lines
- ☐
- ☐

TRIGGER & SYMPTOM NOTES

REMEDIES

(NATURAL)
- ☐ Acupuncture
- ☐ Acupressure
- ☐ Caffeine
- ☐ Dark Room
- ☐ Hot Compress
- ☐ Hydration
- ☐
- ☐
- ☐
- ☐ Ice Pack
- ☐ Massage
- ☐ Relaxation
- ☐ Silence
- ☐ Walk
- ☐
- ☐
- ☐
- ☐

(OTC- COUNTER MEDS)
- ☐ Excedrin
- ☐ Ibuprofen
- ☐ Tylenol
- ☐
- ☐
- ☐
- ☐
- ☐
- ☐

(Rx - PREVENTIVE)
- ☐ Amitriptyline
- ☐ Atenolol
- ☐ Gabapentin
- ☐ Nurtriptyline
- ☐ Propranolol
- ☐ Topamax
- ☐ Valproate
- ☐
- ☐

(Rx - RELIEF)
- ☐ Naproxin
- ☐ Nurtec
- ☐ Sumatriptan
- ☐ Rizatriptan
- ☐ Ubrelvy
- ☐
- ☐

(SUPPLEMENTS)
- ☐ B2
- ☐ Butterbur
- ☐ Feverfew
- ☐ Magnesium
- ☐
- ☐
- ☐

WITHIN 1 HR OF PAIN YES NO   PAIN RELIEF YES NO

REMEDY NOTES

IMPACT ON DAILY ACTIVITIES
NONE | MILD | MODERATE | SEVERE

WWW.ONEMINUTEMIGRAINEDIARY.COM

One Minute **MIGRAINE** Diary

Date : ________________

Start Time : ________________ End Time : ________________ Duration : ________

PAIN SCALE [1-10]

|-----|-----|-----|-----|-----|-----|-----|-----|-----|
1 2 3 4 5 6 7 8 9 10
MILD MODERATE SEVERE

MENSTRUAL PERIOD
YES NO
Birth Control Pills
YES NO

PAIN TYPE
Stabbing Burning Pulsating Shocking Pressure Pounding

SLEEP

WATER

MISSED MEALS
YES NO

PAIN LOCATION
FRONT BACK LEFT RIGHT TOP

WEATHER
TEMP °

STRESS
YES NO

LIGHTS
YES NO

SOUNDS
YES NO

SMELLS
YES NO

FOODS CONSUMED
(within last 24 hours)
- ☐ Alcohol
- ☐ Artificial Sweetener
- ☐ Beans
- ☐ Caffeine
- ☐ Cheese
- ☐ Chocolate
- ☐ Fermented Foods
- ☐ MSG
- ☐ Non Friendly Fruits
- ☐ Nuts
- ☐ Processed Meats
- ☐
- ☐
- ☐

PRODROME
(1-2 hours before headache)
- ☐ Excessive Thirst
- ☐ Excessive Yawning
- ☐ Face Sensitivity
- ☐ Irritability
- ☐ Light Sensitivity
- ☐ Neck Tightness
- ☐ Unexplained Fatigue
- ☐ Visual Disturbances
- ☐
- ☐
- ☐
- ☐
- ☐

SYMPTOMS
- ☐ Distorted Vision
- ☐ Dizziness
- ☐ Irritability
- ☐ Light-headedness
- ☐ Light Sensitivity
- ☐ Malaise
- ☐ Nasal Congestion
- ☐ Nausea/Vomiting
- ☐ Sound Sensitivity
- ☐ Tender Scalp
- ☐
- ☐
- ☐

AURA
(20-30 mins before)
- ☐ Black Spots
- ☐ Flashing Lights
- ☐ Lack of Vision
- ☐ Numbness FACE ARM LEG
- ☐ Zig Zag Lines
- ☐
- ☐

TRIGGER & SYMPTOM NOTES

REMEDIES

(NATURAL)
- ☐ Acupuncture
- ☐ Acupressure
- ☐ Caffeine
- ☐ Dark Room
- ☐ Hot Compress
- ☐ Hydration
- ☐
- ☐
- ☐
- ☐ Ice Pack
- ☐ Massage
- ☐ Relaxation
- ☐ Silence
- ☐ Walk
- ☐
- ☐
- ☐
- ☐

(OTC- COUNTER MEDS)
- ☐ Excedrin
- ☐ Ibuprofen
- ☐ Tylenol
- ☐
- ☐
- ☐
- ☐
- ☐
- ☐

(Rx - PREVENTIVE)
- ☐ Amitriptyline
- ☐ Atenolol
- ☐ Gabapentin
- ☐ Nurtriptyline
- ☐ Propranolol
- ☐ Topamax
- ☐ Valproate
- ☐
- ☐

(Rx - RELIEF)
- ☐ Naproxin
- ☐ Nurtec
- ☐ Sumatriptan
- ☐ Rizatriptan
- ☐ Ubrelvy
- ☐
- ☐

(SUPPLEMENTS)
- ☐ B2
- ☐ Butterbur
- ☐ Feverfew
- ☐ Magnesium
- ☐
- ☐
- ☐

WITHIN 1 HR OF PAIN YES NO PAIN RELIEF YES NO

REMEDY NOTES

IMPACT ON DAILY ACTIVITIES
NONE | MILD | MODERATE | SEVERE

WWW.ONEMINUTEMIGRAINEDIARY.COM

One Minute MIGRAINE Diary

Date : ____________________

Start Time : ____________ End Time : ____________ Duration : ________

PAIN SCALE [1-10]

1 2 3 4 5 6 7 8 9 10

MILD MODERATE SEVERE

MENSTRUAL PERIOD

YES NO

Birth Control Pills

YES NO

PAIN TYPE

Stabbing Burning Pulsating Shocking Pressure Pounding

SLEEP

WATER

MISSED MEALS

YES NO

PAIN LOCATION

FRONT BACK LEFT RIGHT TOP

WEATHER

TEMP °

STRESS

YES NO

LIGHTS

YES NO

SOUNDS

YES NO

SMELLS

YES NO

FOODS CONSUMED (within last 24 hours)

- ☐ Alcohol
- ☐ Artificial Sweetener
- ☐ Beans
- ☐ Caffeine
- ☐ Cheese
- ☐ Chocolate
- ☐ Fermented Foods
- ☐ MSG
- ☐ Non Friendly Fruits
- ☐ Nuts
- ☐ Processed Meats
- ☐
- ☐
- ☐

PRODROME (1-2 hours before headache)

- ☐ Excessive Thirst
- ☐ Excessive Yawning
- ☐ Face Sensitivity
- ☐ Irritability
- ☐ Light Sensitivity
- ☐ Neck Tightness
- ☐ Unexplained Fatigue
- ☐ Visual Disturbances
- ☐
- ☐
- ☐
- ☐
- ☐

SYMPTOMS

- ☐ Distorted Vision
- ☐ Dizziness
- ☐ Irritability
- ☐ Light-headedness
- ☐ Light Sensitivity
- ☐ Malaise
- ☐ Nasal Congestion
- ☐ Nausea/Vomiting
- ☐ Sound Sensitivity
- ☐ Tender Scalp
- ☐
- ☐
- ☐

AURA (20-30 mins before)

- ☐ Black Spots
- ☐ Flashing Lights
- ☐ Lack of Vision
- ☐ Numbness FACE ARM LEG
- ☐ Zig Zag Lines
- ☐
- ☐

TRIGGER & SYMPTOM NOTES

REMEDIES

(NATURAL)

- ☐ Acupuncture
- ☐ Ice Pack
- ☐ Acupressure
- ☐ Massage
- ☐ Caffeine
- ☐ Relaxation
- ☐ Dark Room
- ☐ Silence
- ☐ Hot Compress
- ☐ Walk
- ☐ Hydration
- ☐
- ☐
- ☐
- ☐
- ☐
- ☐
- ☐

(OTC- COUNTER MEDS)

- ☐ Excedrin
- ☐ Ibuprofen
- ☐ Tylenol
- ☐
- ☐
- ☐
- ☐
- ☐
- ☐

(Rx - PREVENTIVE)

- ☐ Amitriptyline
- ☐ Atenolol
- ☐ Gabapentin
- ☐ Nurtriptyline
- ☐ Propranolol
- ☐ Topamax
- ☐ Valproate
- ☐
- ☐

(Rx - RELIEF)

- ☐ Naproxin
- ☐ Nurtec
- ☐ Sumatriptan
- ☐ Rizatriptan
- ☐ Ubrelvy
- ☐
- ☐

(SUPPLEMENTS)

- ☐ B2
- ☐ Butterbur
- ☐ Feverfew
- ☐ Magnesium
- ☐
- ☐
- ☐

WITHIN 1 HR OF PAIN YES NO PAIN RELIEF YES NO

REMEDY NOTES

IMPACT ON DAILY ACTIVITIES

NONE | MILD | MODERATE | SEVERE

WWW.ONEMINUTEMIGRAINEDIARY.COM

One Minute MIGRAINE Diary

Date : ______________________

Start Time : ______________ End Time : ______________ Duration : ________

PAIN SCALE [1-10]

1 2 3 4 5 6 7 8 9 10

MILD MODERATE SEVERE

MENSTRUAL PERIOD

YES NO

Birth Control Pills

YES NO

PAIN TYPE

Stabbing Burning Pulsating Shocking Pressure Pounding

SLEEP

WATER

MISSED MEALS

YES NO

PAIN LOCATION

FRONT BACK LEFT RIGHT TOP

WEATHER

TEMP °

STRESS

YES NO

LIGHTS

YES NO

SOUNDS

YES NO

SMELLS

YES NO

FOODS CONSUMED (within last 24 hours)

- ☐ Alcohol
- ☐ Artificial Sweetener
- ☐ Beans
- ☐ Caffeine
- ☐ Cheese
- ☐ Chocolate
- ☐ Fermented Foods
- ☐ MSG
- ☐ Non Friendly Fruits
- ☐ Nuts
- ☐ Processed Meats
- ☐
- ☐
- ☐

PRODROME (1-2 hours before headache)

- ☐ Excessive Thirst
- ☐ Excessive Yawning
- ☐ Face Sensitivity
- ☐ Irritability
- ☐ Light Sensitivity
- ☐ Neck Tightness
- ☐ Unexplained Fatigue
- ☐ Visual Disturbances
- ☐
- ☐
- ☐
- ☐
- ☐

SYMPTOMS

- ☐ Distorted Vision
- ☐ Dizziness
- ☐ Irritability
- ☐ Light-headedness
- ☐ Light Sensitivity
- ☐ Malaise
- ☐ Nasal Congestion
- ☐ Nausea/Vomiting
- ☐ Sound Sensitivity
- ☐ Tender Scalp
- ☐
- ☐
- ☐

AURA (20-30 mins before)

- ☐ Black Spots
- ☐ Flashing Lights
- ☐ Lack of Vision
- ☐ Numbness FACE ARM LEG
- ☐ Zig Zag Lines
- ☐
- ☐

TRIGGER & SYMPTOM NOTES

REMEDIES

(NATURAL)

- ☐ Acupuncture
- ☐ Acupressure
- ☐ Caffeine
- ☐ Dark Room
- ☐ Hot Compress
- ☐ Hydration
- ☐
- ☐
- ☐
- ☐ Ice Pack
- ☐ Massage
- ☐ Relaxation
- ☐ Silence
- ☐ Walk
- ☐
- ☐
- ☐
- ☐

(OTC- COUNTER MEDS)

- ☐ Excedrin
- ☐ Ibuprofen
- ☐ Tylenol
- ☐
- ☐
- ☐
- ☐
- ☐
- ☐

(Rx - PREVENTIVE)

- ☐ Amitriptyline
- ☐ Atenolol
- ☐ Gabapentin
- ☐ Nurtriptyline
- ☐ Propranolol
- ☐ Topamax
- ☐ Valproate
- ☐
- ☐

(Rx - RELIEF)

- ☐ Naproxin
- ☐ Nurtec
- ☐ Sumatriptan
- ☐ Rizatriptan
- ☐ Ubrelvy
- ☐
- ☐

(SUPPLEMENTS)

- ☐ B2
- ☐ Butterbur
- ☐ Feverfew
- ☐ Magnesium
- ☐
- ☐
- ☐

WITHIN 1 HR OF PAIN YES NO PAIN RELIEF YES NO

REMEDY NOTES

IMPACT ON DAILY ACTIVITIES

NONE | MILD | MODERATE | SEVERE

WWW.ONEMINUTEMIGRAINEDIARY.COM

One Minute MIGRAINE Diary

Date : ______________________

Start Time : ______________ End Time : ______________ Duration : ________

PAIN SCALE [1-10]

1 2 3 4 5 6 7 8 9 10

MILD MODERATE SEVERE

MENSTRUAL PERIOD

YES NO

Birth Control Pills

YES NO

PAIN TYPE

Stabbing Burning Pulsating Shocking Pressure Pounding

SLEEP

WATER

MISSED MEALS

YES NO

PAIN LOCATION

FRONT BACK LEFT RIGHT TOP

WEATHER

TEMP °

STRESS

YES NO

LIGHTS

YES NO

SOUNDS

YES NO

SMELLS

YES NO

FOODS CONSUMED (within last 24 hours)

- ☐ Alcohol
- ☐ Artificial Sweetener
- ☐ Beans
- ☐ Caffeine
- ☐ Cheese
- ☐ Chocolate
- ☐ Fermented Foods
- ☐ MSG
- ☐ Non Friendly Fruits
- ☐ Nuts
- ☐ Processed Meats
- ☐
- ☐
- ☐

PRODROME (1-2 hours before headache)

- ☐ Excessive Thirst
- ☐ Excessive Yawning
- ☐ Face Sensitivity
- ☐ Irritability
- ☐ Light Sensitivity
- ☐ Neck Tightness
- ☐ Unexplained Fatigue
- ☐ Visual Disturbances
- ☐
- ☐
- ☐
- ☐
- ☐

SYMPTOMS

- ☐ Distorted Vision
- ☐ Dizziness
- ☐ Irritability
- ☐ Light-headedness
- ☐ Light Sensitivity
- ☐ Malaise
- ☐ Nasal Congestion
- ☐ Nausea/Vomiting
- ☐ Sound Sensitivity
- ☐ Tender Scalp
- ☐
- ☐
- ☐

AURA (20-30 mins before)

- ☐ Black Spots
- ☐ Flashing Lights
- ☐ Lack of Vision
- ☐ Numbness FACE ARM LEG
- ☐ Zig Zag Lines
- ☐
- ☐

TRIGGER & SYMPTOM NOTES

REMEDIES

(NATURAL)

- ☐ Acupuncture
- ☐ Acupressure
- ☐ Caffeine
- ☐ Dark Room
- ☐ Hot Compress
- ☐ Hydration
- ☐
- ☐
- ☐
- ☐ Ice Pack
- ☐ Massage
- ☐ Relaxation
- ☐ Silence
- ☐ Walk
- ☐
- ☐
- ☐
- ☐

(OTC- COUNTER MEDS)

- ☐ Excedrin
- ☐ Ibuprofen
- ☐ Tylenol
- ☐
- ☐
- ☐
- ☐
- ☐
- ☐

(Rx - PREVENTIVE)

- ☐ Amitriptyline
- ☐ Atenolol
- ☐ Gabapentin
- ☐ Nurtriptyline
- ☐ Propranolol
- ☐ Topamax
- ☐ Valproate
- ☐
- ☐

(Rx - RELIEF)

- ☐ Naproxin
- ☐ Nurtec
- ☐ Sumatriptan
- ☐ Rizatriptan
- ☐ Ubrelvy
- ☐
- ☐

(SUPPLEMENTS)

- ☐ B2
- ☐ Butterbur
- ☐ Feverfew
- ☐ Magnesium
- ☐
- ☐
- ☐

WITHIN 1 HR OF PAIN YES NO PAIN RELIEF YES NO

REMEDY NOTES

IMPACT ON DAILY ACTIVITIES

NONE | MILD | MODERATE | SEVERE

WWW.ONEMINUTEMIGRAINEDIARY.COM

One Minute MIGRAINE Diary

Date : ____________________

Start Time : ____________________ End Time : ________________ Duration : ________

PAIN SCALE [1-10]
1 2 3 4 5 6 7 8 9 10
MILD MODERATE SEVERE

MENSTRUAL PERIOD
YES NO
Birth Control Pills
YES NO

PAIN TYPE
Stabbing Burning Pulsating Shocking Pressure Pounding

SLEEP

WATER

MISSED MEALS
YES NO

PAIN LOCATION
FRONT BACK LEFT RIGHT TOP

WEATHER
TEMP °

STRESS
YES NO

LIGHTS
YES NO

SOUNDS
YES NO

SMELLS
YES NO

FOODS CONSUMED (within last 24 hours)	PRODROME (1-2 hours before headache)	SYMPTOMS	AURA (20-30 mins before)
☐ Alcohol	☐ Excessive Thirst	☐ Distorted Vision	☐ Black Spots
☐ Artificial Sweetener	☐ Excessive Yawning	☐ Dizziness	☐ Flashing Lights
☐ Beans	☐ Face Sensitivity	☐ Irritability	☐ Lack of Vision
☐ Caffeine	☐ Irritability	☐ Light-headedness	☐ Numbness FACE ARM LEG
☐ Cheese	☐ Light Sensitivity	☐ Light Sensitivity	☐ Zig Zag Lines
☐ Chocolate	☐ Neck Tightness	☐ Malaise	☐
☐ Fermented Foods	☐ Unexplained Fatigue	☐ Nasal Congestion	☐
☐ MSG	☐ Visual Disturbances	☐ Nausea/Vomiting	**TRIGGER & SYMPTOM NOTES**
☐ Non Friendly Fruits	☐	☐ Sound Sensitivity	
☐ Nuts	☐	☐ Tender Scalp	
☐ Processed Meats	☐	☐	
☐	☐	☐	
☐	☐	☐	
☐	☐		

REMEDIES

(NATURAL)		(OTC- COUNTER MEDS)	(Rx - PREVENTIVE)	(Rx - RELIEF)	(SUPPLEMENTS)
☐ Acupuncture	☐ Ice Pack	☐ Excedrin	☐ Amitriptyline	☐ Naproxin	☐ B2
☐ Acupressure	☐ Massage	☐ Ibuprofen	☐ Atenolol	☐ Nurtec	☐ Butterbur
☐ Caffeine	☐ Relaxation	☐ Tylenol	☐ Gabapentin	☐ Sumatriptan	☐ Feverfew
☐ Dark Room	☐ Silence	☐	☐ Nurtriptyline	☐ Rizatriptan	☐ Magnesium
☐ Hot Compress	☐ Walk	☐	☐ Propranolol	☐ Ubrelvy	☐
☐ Hydration	☐	☐	☐ Topamax	☐	☐
☐	☐	☐	☐ Valproate	☐	☐
☐	☐	☐	☐	WITHIN 1 HR OF PAIN YES NO	PAIN RELIEF YES NO
☐	☐	☐	☐		

REMEDY NOTES

IMPACT ON DAILY ACTIVITIES
NONE | MILD | MODERATE | SEVERE

WWW.ONEMINUTEMIGRAINEDIARY.COM

One Minute MIGRAINE Diary

Date : ______________________

Start Time : ______________ End Time : ____________ Duration : ______

PAIN SCALE [1-10]	MENSTRUAL PERIOD	PAIN TYPE	WATER
1 2 3 4 5 6 7 8 9 10 MILD MODERATE SEVERE	YES NO Birth Control Pills YES NO	Stabbing Burning Pulsating Shocking Pressure Pounding **SLEEP**	**MISSED MEALS** YES NO
PAIN LOCATION FRONT BACK LEFT RIGHT TOP		**WEATHER** TEMP °	**STRESS** YES NO
		LIGHTS YES NO **SOUNDS** YES NO	**SMELLS** YES NO

FOODS CONSUMED (within last 24 hours)	PRODROME (1-2 hours before headache)	SYMPTOMS	AURA (20-30 mins before)
☐ Alcohol	☐ Excessive Thirst	☐ Distorted Vision	☐ Black Spots
☐ Artificial Sweetener	☐ Excessive Yawning	☐ Dizziness	☐ Flashing Lights
☐ Beans	☐ Face Sensitivity	☐ Irritability	☐ Lack of Vision
☐ Caffeine	☐ Irritability	☐ Light-headedness	☐ Numbness FACE ARM LEG
☐ Cheese	☐ Light Sensitivity	☐ Light Sensitivity	☐ Zig Zag Lines
☐ Chocolate	☐ Neck Tightness	☐ Malaise	☐
☐ Fermented Foods	☐ Unexplained Fatigue	☐ Nasal Congestion	☐
☐ MSG	☐ Visual Disturbances	☐ Nausea/Vomiting	**TRIGGER & SYMPTOM NOTES**
☐ Non Friendly Fruits	☐	☐ Sound Sensitivity	
☐ Nuts	☐	☐ Tender Scalp	
☐ Processed Meats	☐	☐	
☐	☐	☐	
☐	☐	☐	
☐			

REMEDIES

(NATURAL)		(OTC- COUNTER MEDS)	(Rx - PREVENTIVE)	(Rx - RELIEF)	(SUPPLEMENTS)
☐ Acupuncture	☐ Ice Pack	☐ Excedrin	☐ Amitriptyline	☐ Naproxin	☐ B2
☐ Acupressure	☐ Massage	☐ Ibuprofen	☐ Atenolol	☐ Nurtec	☐ Butterbur
☐ Caffeine	☐ Relaxation	☐ Tylenol	☐ Gabapentin	☐ Sumatriptan	☐ Feverfew
☐ Dark Room	☐ Silence	☐	☐ Nurtriptyline	☐ Rizatriptan	☐ Magnesium
☐ Hot Compress	☐ Walk	☐	☐ Propranolol	☐ Ubrelvy	☐
☐ Hydration	☐	☐	☐ Topamax	☐	☐
☐	☐	☐	☐ Valproate	☐	☐
☐	☐	☐	☐	WITHIN 1 HR OF PAIN YES NO	PAIN RELIEF YES NO
☐	☐	☐	☐		

REMEDY NOTES

IMPACT ON DAILY ACTIVITIES

NONE | MILD | MODERATE | SEVERE

WWW.ONEMINUTEMIGRAINEDIARY.COM

One Minute MIGRAINE Diary

Date : ____________

Start Time : ____________ End Time : ____________ Duration : ________

PAIN SCALE [1-10]	MENSTRUAL PERIOD	PAIN TYPE	WATER
1 2 3 4 5 6 7 8 9 10 MILD MODERATE SEVERE	YES NO Birth Control Pills YES NO	Stabbing Burning Pulsating Shocking Pressure Pounding SLEEP	MISSED MEALS YES NO

PAIN LOCATION	WEATHER	STRESS
FRONT BACK LEFT RIGHT TOP	TEMP °	YES NO
	LIGHTS YES NO / SOUNDS YES NO	SMELLS YES NO

FOODS CONSUMED (within last 24 hours)	PRODROME (1-2 hours before headache)	SYMPTOMS	AURA (20-30 mins before)
☐ Alcohol	☐ Excessive Thirst	☐ Distorted Vision	☐ Black Spots
☐ Artificial Sweetener	☐ Excessive Yawning	☐ Dizziness	☐ Flashing Lights
☐ Beans	☐ Face Sensitivity	☐ Irritability	☐ Lack of Vision
☐ Caffeine	☐ Irritability	☐ Light-headedness	☐ Numbness FACE ARM LEG
☐ Cheese	☐ Light Sensitivity	☐ Light Sensitivity	☐ Zig Zag Lines
☐ Chocolate	☐ Neck Tightness	☐ Malaise	☐
☐ Fermented Foods	☐ Unexplained Fatigue	☐ Nasal Congestion	☐
☐ MSG	☐ Visual Disturbances	☐ Nausea/Vomiting	TRIGGER & SYMPTOM NOTES
☐ Non Friendly Fruits	☐	☐ Sound Sensitivity	
☐ Nuts	☐	☐ Tender Scalp	
☐ Processed Meats	☐	☐	
☐	☐	☐	
☐	☐	☐	
☐	☐		

REMEDIES

(NATURAL)		(OTC- COUNTER MEDS)	(Rx - PREVENTIVE)	(Rx - RELIEF)	(SUPPLEMENTS)
☐ Acupuncture	☐ Ice Pack	☐ Excedrin	☐ Amitriptyline	☐ Naproxin	☐ B2
☐ Acupressure	☐ Massage	☐ Ibuprofen	☐ Atenolol	☐ Nurtec	☐ Butterbur
☐ Caffeine	☐ Relaxation	☐ Tylenol	☐ Gabapentin	☐ Sumatriptan	☐ Feverfew
☐ Dark Room	☐ Silence	☐	☐ Nurtriptyline	☐ Rizatriptan	☐ Magnesium
☐ Hot Compress	☐ Walk	☐	☐ Propranolol	☐ Ubrelvy	☐
☐ Hydration	☐	☐	☐ Topamax	☐	☐
☐	☐	☐	☐ Valproate	☐	☐
☐	☐	☐	☐	WITHIN 1 HR OF PAIN YES NO	PAIN RELIEF YES NO
☐	☐	☐	☐		

REMEDY NOTES

IMPACT ON DAILY ACTIVITIES

NONE | MILD | MODERATE | SEVERE

WWW.ONEMINUTEMIGRAINEDIARY.COM

One Minute MIGRAINE Diary

Date : ______________________

Start Time : ______________ End Time : ______________ Duration : ________

PAIN SCALE [1-10]	MENSTRUAL PERIOD	PAIN TYPE	WATER
1 2 3 4 5 6 7 8 9 10 MILD MODERATE SEVERE	YES NO Birth Control Pills YES NO	Stabbing Burning Pulsating Shocking Pressure Pounding SLEEP	MISSED MEALS YES NO

PAIN LOCATION

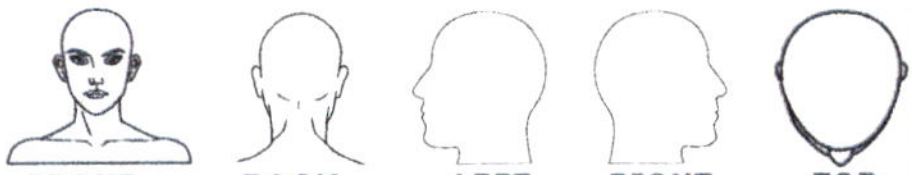

FRONT BACK LEFT RIGHT TOP

WEATHER

TEMP °

LIGHTS YES NO

SOUNDS YES NO

STRESS YES NO

SMELLS YES NO

FOODS CONSUMED (within last 24 hours)	PRODROME (1-2 hours before headache)	SYMPTOMS	AURA (20-30 mins before)
☐ Alcohol	☐ Excessive Thirst	☐ Distorted Vision	☐ Black Spots
☐ Artificial Sweetener	☐ Excessive Yawning	☐ Dizziness	☐ Flashing Lights
☐ Beans	☐ Face Sensitivity	☐ Irritability	☐ Lack of Vision
☐ Caffeine	☐ Irritability	☐ Light-headedness	☐ Numbness FACE ARM LEG
☐ Cheese	☐ Light Sensitivity	☐ Light Sensitivity	☐ Zig Zag Lines
☐ Chocolate	☐ Neck Tightness	☐ Malaise	☐
☐ Fermented Foods	☐ Unexplained Fatigue	☐ Nasal Congestion	☐
☐ MSG	☐ Visual Disturbances	☐ Nausea/Vomiting	TRIGGER & SYMPTOM NOTES
☐ Non Friendly Fruits	☐	☐ Sound Sensitivity	
☐ Nuts	☐	☐ Tender Scalp	
☐ Processed Meats	☐	☐	
☐	☐	☐	
☐	☐	☐	
☐			

REMEDIES

(NATURAL)		(OTC- COUNTER MEDS)	(Rx - PREVENTIVE)	(Rx - RELIEF)	(SUPPLEMENTS)
☐ Acupuncture	☐ Ice Pack	☐ Excedrin	☐ Amitriptyline	☐ Naproxin	☐ B2
☐ Acupressure	☐ Massage	☐ Ibuprofen	☐ Atenolol	☐ Nurtec	☐ Butterbur
☐ Caffeine	☐ Relaxation	☐ Tylenol	☐ Gabapentin	☐ Sumatriptan	☐ Feverfew
☐ Dark Room	☐ Silence	☐	☐ Nurtriptyline	☐ Rizatriptan	☐ Magnesium
☐ Hot Compress	☐ Walk	☐	☐ Propranolol	☐ Ubrelvy	☐
☐ Hydration	☐	☐	☐ Topamax	☐	☐
☐	☐	☐	☐ Valproate	☐	☐
☐	☐	☐	☐	WITHIN 1 HR OF PAIN YES NO	PAIN RELIEF YES NO
☐	☐	☐	☐		

REMEDY NOTES

IMPACT ON DAILY ACTIVITIES

NONE | MILD | MODERATE | SEVERE

WWW.ONEMINUTEMIGRAINEDIARY.COM

One Minute
MIGRAINE Diary

Date : ____________________

Start Time : ____________________ End Time : ____________________ Duration : __________

PAIN SCALE [1-10]

|-----|-----|-----|-----|-----|-----|-----|-----|-----|
1 2 3 4 5 6 7 8 9 10
MILD MODERATE SEVERE

MENSTRUAL PERIOD
YES NO
Birth Control Pills
YES NO

PAIN TYPE
Stabbing Burning Pulsating Shocking Pressure Pounding

SLEEP

WATER

MISSED MEALS
YES NO

PAIN LOCATION

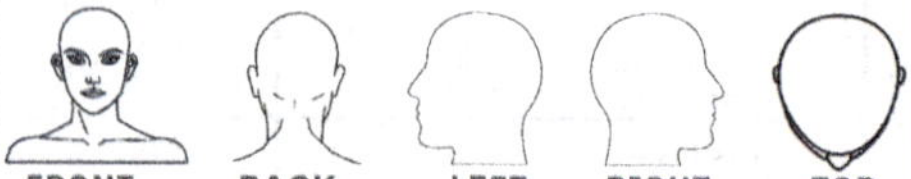

FRONT BACK LEFT RIGHT TOP

WEATHER
° TEMP

STRESS
YES NO

LIGHTS
YES NO

SOUNDS
YES NO

SMELLS
YES NO

FOODS CONSUMED (within last 24 hours)	PRODROME (1-2 hours before headache)	SYMPTOMS	AURA (20-30 mins before)
☐ Alcohol	☐ Excessive Thirst	☐ Distorted Vision	☐ Black Spots
☐ Artificial Sweetener	☐ Excessive Yawning	☐ Dizziness	☐ Flashing Lights
☐ Beans	☐ Face Sensitivity	☐ Irritability	☐ Lack of Vision
☐ Caffeine	☐ Irritability	☐ Light-headedness	☐ Numbness FACE ARM LEG
☐ Cheese	☐ Light Sensitivity	☐ Light Sensitivity	☐ Zig Zag Lines
☐ Chocolate	☐ Neck Tightness	☐ Malaise	☐
☐ Fermented Foods	☐ Unexplained Fatigue	☐ Nasal Congestion	☐
☐ MSG	☐ Visual Disturbances	☐ Nausea/Vomiting	TRIGGER & SYMPTOM NOTES
☐ Non Friendly Fruits	☐	☐ Sound Sensitivity	
☐ Nuts	☐	☐ Tender Scalp	
☐ Processed Meats	☐	☐	
☐	☐	☐	
☐	☐	☐	
☐			

REMEDIES

(NATURAL)		(OTC- COUNTER MEDS)	(Rx - PREVENTIVE)	(Rx - RELIEF)	(SUPPLEMENTS)
☐ Acupuncture	☐ Ice Pack	☐ Excedrin	☐ Amitriptyline	☐ Naproxin	☐ B2
☐ Acupressure	☐ Massage	☐ Ibuprofen	☐ Atenolol	☐ Nurtec	☐ Butterbur
☐ Caffeine	☐ Relaxation	☐ Tylenol	☐ Gabapentin	☐ Sumatriptan	☐ Feverfew
☐ Dark Room	☐ Silence	☐	☐ Nurtriptyline	☐ Rizatriptan	☐ Magnesium
☐ Hot Compress	☐ Walk	☐	☐ Propranolol	☐ Ubrelvy	☐
☐ Hydration	☐	☐	☐ Topamax	☐	☐
☐	☐	☐	☐ Valproate	☐	☐
☐	☐	☐	☐	WITHIN 1 HR OF PAIN YES NO	PAIN RELIEF YES NO
☐	☐	☐	☐		

REMEDY NOTES

IMPACT ON DAILY ACTIVITIES
NONE | MILD | MODERATE | SEVERE

WWW.ONEMINUTEMIGRAINEDIARY.COM

One Minute MIGRAINE Diary

Date : ______________________

Start Time : ______________ End Time : ______________ Duration : ________

PAIN SCALE [1-10]

1 2 3 4 5 6 7 8 9 10

MILD MODERATE SEVERE

MENSTRUAL PERIOD

YES NO

Birth Control Pills

YES NO

PAIN TYPE

Stabbing Burning Pulsating Shocking Pressure Pounding

SLEEP

WATER

MISSED MEALS

YES NO

PAIN LOCATION

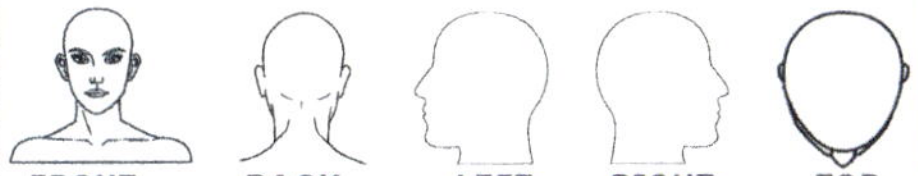

FRONT BACK LEFT RIGHT TOP

WEATHER

TEMP °

STRESS

YES NO

LIGHTS

YES NO

SOUNDS

YES NO

SMELLS

YES NO

FOODS CONSUMED (within last 24 hours)	PRODROME (1-2 hours before headache)	SYMPTOMS	AURA (20-30 mins before)
☐ Alcohol	☐ Excessive Thirst	☐ Distorted Vision	☐ Black Spots
☐ Artificial Sweetener	☐ Excessive Yawning	☐ Dizziness	☐ Flashing Lights
☐ Beans	☐ Face Sensitivity	☐ Irritability	☐ Lack of Vision
☐ Caffeine	☐ Irritability	☐ Light-headedness	☐ Numbness FACE ARM LEG
☐ Cheese	☐ Light Sensitivity	☐ Light Sensitivity	☐ Zig Zag Lines
☐ Chocolate	☐ Neck Tightness	☐ Malaise	☐
☐ Fermented Foods	☐ Unexplained Fatigue	☐ Nasal Congestion	☐
☐ MSG	☐ Visual Disturbances	☐ Nausea/Vomiting	**TRIGGER & SYMPTOM NOTES**
☐ Non Friendly Fruits	☐	☐ Sound Sensitivity	
☐ Nuts	☐	☐ Tender Scalp	
☐ Processed Meats	☐	☐	
☐	☐	☐	
☐	☐	☐	
☐	☐		

REMEDIES

(NATURAL)		(OTC- COUNTER MEDS)	(Rx - PREVENTIVE)	(Rx - RELIEF)	(SUPPLEMENTS)
☐ Acupuncture	☐ Ice Pack	☐ Excedrin	☐ Amitriptyline	☐ Naproxin	☐ B2
☐ Acupressure	☐ Massage	☐ Ibuprofen	☐ Atenolol	☐ Nurtec	☐ Butterbur
☐ Caffeine	☐ Relaxation	☐ Tylenol	☐ Gabapentin	☐ Sumatriptan	☐ Feverfew
☐ Dark Room	☐ Silence	☐	☐ Nurtriptyline	☐ Rizatriptan	☐ Magnesium
☐ Hot Compress	☐ Walk	☐	☐ Propranolol	☐ Ubrelvy	☐
☐ Hydration	☐	☐	☐ Topamax	☐	☐
☐	☐	☐	☐ Valproate	☐	☐
☐	☐	☐	☐	WITHIN 1 HR OF PAIN YES NO	PAIN RELIEF YES NO
☐	☐	☐	☐		

REMEDY NOTES

IMPACT ON DAILY ACTIVITIES

NONE | MILD | MODERATE | SEVERE

WWW.ONEMINUTEMIGRAINEDIARY.COM

One Minute MIGRAINE Diary

Date : ____________________

Start Time : ______________ End Time : ______________ Duration : ________

PAIN SCALE [1-10]

1 2 3 4 5 6 7 8 9 10

MILD MODERATE SEVERE

MENSTRUAL PERIOD

YES NO

Birth Control Pills

YES NO

PAIN TYPE

Stabbing Burning Pulsating Shocking Pressure Pounding

SLEEP

WATER

MISSED MEALS

YES NO

PAIN LOCATION

FRONT BACK LEFT RIGHT TOP

WEATHER

TEMP °

STRESS

YES NO

LIGHTS

YES NO

SOUNDS

YES NO

SMELLS

YES NO

FOODS CONSUMED (within last 24 hours)	PRODROME (1-2 hours before headache)	SYMPTOMS	AURA (20-30 mins before)
☐ Alcohol	☐ Excessive Thirst	☐ Distorted Vision	☐ Black Spots
☐ Artificial Sweetener	☐ Excessive Yawning	☐ Dizziness	☐ Flashing Lights
☐ Beans	☐ Face Sensitivity	☐ Irritability	☐ Lack of Vision
☐ Caffeine	☐ Irritability	☐ Light-headedness	☐ Numbness FACE ARM LEG
☐ Cheese	☐ Light Sensitivity	☐ Light Sensitivity	☐ Zig Zag Lines
☐ Chocolate	☐ Neck Tightness	☐ Malaise	☐
☐ Fermented Foods	☐ Unexplained Fatigue	☐ Nasal Congestion	☐
☐ MSG	☐ Visual Disturbances	☐ Nausea/Vomiting	TRIGGER & SYMPTOM NOTES
☐ Non Friendly Fruits	☐	☐ Sound Sensitivity	
☐ Nuts	☐	☐ Tender Scalp	
☐ Processed Meats	☐	☐	
☐	☐	☐	
☐	☐	☐	
☐	☐		

REMEDIES

(NATURAL)		(OTC- COUNTER MEDS)	(Rx - PREVENTIVE)	(Rx - RELIEF)	(SUPPLEMENTS)
☐ Acupuncture	☐ Ice Pack	☐ Excedrin	☐ Amitriptyline	☐ Naproxin	☐ B2
☐ Acupressure	☐ Massage	☐ Ibuprofen	☐ Atenolol	☐ Nurtec	☐ Butterbur
☐ Caffeine	☐ Relaxation	☐ Tylenol	☐ Gabapentin	☐ Sumatriptan	☐ Feverfew
☐ Dark Room	☐ Silence	☐	☐ Nurtriptyline	☐ Rizatriptan	☐ Magnesium
☐ Hot Compress	☐ Walk	☐	☐ Propranolol	☐ Ubrelvy	☐
☐ Hydration	☐	☐	☐ Topamax	☐	☐
☐	☐	☐	☐ Valproate	☐	☐
☐	☐	☐	☐	WITHIN 1 HR OF PAIN YES NO	PAIN RELIEF YES NO
☐	☐	☐	☐		

REMEDY NOTES

IMPACT ON DAILY ACTIVITIES

NONE | MILD | MODERATE | SEVERE

WWW.ONEMINUTEMIGRAINEDIARY.COM

One Minute MIGRAINE Diary

Date :

Start Time : End Time : Duration :

PAIN SCALE [1-10]	MENSTRUAL PERIOD	PAIN TYPE	WATER
1 2 3 4 5 6 7 8 9 10 MILD MODERATE SEVERE	YES NO Birth Control Pills YES NO	Stabbing Burning Pulsating Shocking Pressure Pounding SLEEP	MISSED MEALS YES NO

PAIN LOCATION	WEATHER	STRESS
FRONT BACK LEFT RIGHT TOP	° TEMP	YES NO
	LIGHTS YES NO SOUNDS YES NO	SMELLS YES NO

FOODS CONSUMED (within last 24 hours)	PRODROME (1-2 hours before headache)	SYMPTOMS	AURA (20-30 mins before)
☐ Alcohol	☐ Excessive Thirst	☐ Distorted Vision	☐ Black Spots
☐ Artificial Sweetener	☐ Excessive Yawning	☐ Dizziness	☐ Flashing Lights
☐ Beans	☐ Face Sensitivity	☐ Irritability	☐ Lack of Vision
☐ Caffeine	☐ Irritability	☐ Light-headedness	☐ Numbness FACE ARM LEG
☐ Cheese	☐ Light Sensitivity	☐ Light Sensitivity	☐ Zig Zag Lines
☐ Chocolate	☐ Neck Tightness	☐ Malaise	☐
☐ Fermented Foods	☐ Unexplained Fatigue	☐ Nasal Congestion	☐
☐ MSG	☐ Visual Disturbances	☐ Nausea/Vomiting	TRIGGER & SYMPTOM NOTES
☐ Non Friendly Fruits	☐	☐ Sound Sensitivity	
☐ Nuts	☐	☐ Tender Scalp	
☐ Processed Meats	☐	☐	
☐	☐	☐	
☐	☐	☐	
☐	☐		

REMEDIES

(NATURAL)		(OTC- COUNTER MEDS)	(Rx - PREVENTIVE)	(Rx - RELIEF)	(SUPPLEMENTS)
☐ Acupuncture	☐ Ice Pack	☐ Excedrin	☐ Amitriptyline	☐ Naproxin	☐ B2
☐ Acupressure	☐ Massage	☐ Ibuprofen	☐ Atenolol	☐ Nurtec	☐ Butterbur
☐ Caffeine	☐ Relaxation	☐ Tylenol	☐ Gabapentin	☐ Sumatriptan	☐ Feverfew
☐ Dark Room	☐ Silence	☐	☐ Nurtriptyline	☐ Rizatriptan	☐ Magnesium
☐ Hot Compress	☐ Walk	☐	☐ Propranolol	☐ Ubrelvy	☐
☐ Hydration	☐	☐	☐ Topamax	☐	☐
☐	☐	☐	☐ Valproate	☐	☐
☐	☐	☐	☐	WITHIN 1 HR OF PAIN YES NO	PAIN RELIEF YES NO
☐	☐	☐	☐		

REMEDY NOTES

IMPACT ON DAILY ACTIVITIES

NONE | MILD | MODERATE | SEVERE

WWW.ONEMINUTEMIGRAINEDIARY.COM

One Minute MIGRAINE Diary

Date : ______________________

Start Time : ______________ End Time : ____________ Duration : ________

PAIN SCALE [1-10]

1 2 3 4 5 6 7 8 9 10

MILD MODERATE SEVERE

MENSTRUAL PERIOD

YES NO

Birth Control Pills

YES NO

PAIN TYPE

Stabbing Burning Pulsating Shocking Pressure Pounding

SLEEP

WATER

MISSED MEALS

YES NO

PAIN LOCATION

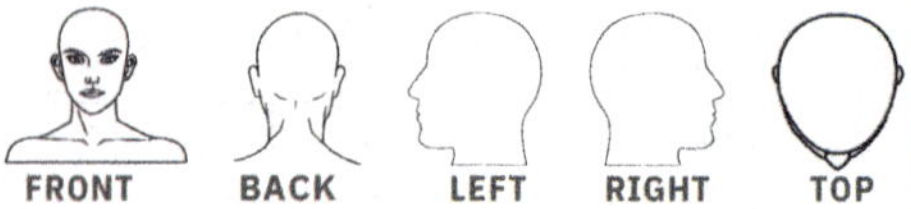

FRONT BACK LEFT RIGHT TOP

WEATHER

° TEMP

STRESS

YES NO

LIGHTS

YES NO

SOUNDS

YES NO

SMELLS

YES NO

FOODS CONSUMED (within last 24 hours)	PRODROME (1-2 hours before headache)	SYMPTOMS	AURA (20-30 mins before)
☐ Alcohol	☐ Excessive Thirst	☐ Distorted Vision	☐ Black Spots
☐ Artificial Sweetener	☐ Excessive Yawning	☐ Dizziness	☐ Flashing Lights
☐ Beans	☐ Face Sensitivity	☐ Irritability	☐ Lack of Vision
☐ Caffeine	☐ Irritability	☐ Light-headedness	☐ Numbness FACE ARM LEG
☐ Cheese	☐ Light Sensitivity	☐ Light Sensitivity	☐ Zig Zag Lines
☐ Chocolate	☐ Neck Tightness	☐ Malaise	☐
☐ Fermented Foods	☐ Unexplained Fatigue	☐ Nasal Congestion	☐
☐ MSG	☐ Visual Disturbances	☐ Nausea/Vomiting	TRIGGER & SYMPTOM NOTES
☐ Non Friendly Fruits	☐	☐ Sound Sensitivity	
☐ Nuts	☐	☐ Tender Scalp	
☐ Processed Meats	☐	☐	
☐	☐	☐	
☐	☐	☐	
☐			

REMEDIES

(NATURAL)		(OTC- COUNTER MEDS)	(Rx - PREVENTIVE)	(Rx - RELIEF)	(SUPPLEMENTS)
☐ Acupuncture	☐ Ice Pack	☐ Excedrin	☐ Amitriptyline	☐ Naproxin	☐ B2
☐ Acupressure	☐ Massage	☐ Ibuprofen	☐ Atenolol	☐ Nurtec	☐ Butterbur
☐ Caffeine	☐ Relaxation	☐ Tylenol	☐ Gabapentin	☐ Sumatriptan	☐ Feverfew
☐ Dark Room	☐ Silence	☐	☐ Nurtriptyline	☐ Rizatriptan	☐ Magnesium
☐ Hot Compress	☐ Walk	☐	☐ Propranolol	☐ Ubrelvy	☐
☐ Hydration	☐	☐	☐ Topamax	☐	☐
☐	☐	☐	☐ Valproate	☐	☐
☐	☐	☐	☐	WITHIN 1 HR OF PAIN YES NO	PAIN RELIEF YES NO
☐	☐	☐	☐		

REMEDY NOTES

IMPACT ON DAILY ACTIVITIES

NONE | MILD | MODERATE | SEVERE

WWW.ONEMINUTEMIGRAINEDIARY.COM

One Minute MIGRAINE Diary

Date : ______________________

Start Time : ______________ End Time : ____________ Duration : ________

PAIN SCALE [1-10]

1 2 3 4 5 6 7 8 9 10

MILD MODERATE SEVERE

MENSTRUAL PERIOD

YES NO

Birth Control Pills

YES NO

PAIN TYPE

Stabbing Burning Pulsating Shocking Pressure Pounding

SLEEP

WATER

MISSED MEALS

YES NO

PAIN LOCATION

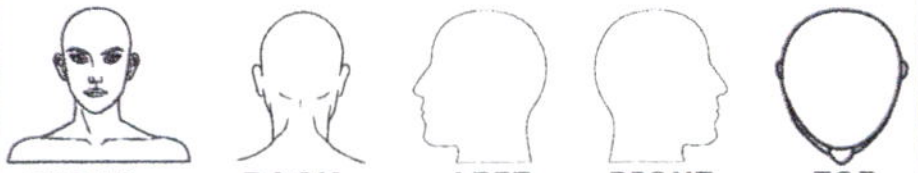

FRONT BACK LEFT RIGHT TOP

WEATHER

TEMP °

STRESS

YES NO

LIGHTS

YES NO

SOUNDS

YES NO

SMELLS

YES NO

FOODS CONSUMED (within last 24 hours)	PRODROME (1-2 hours before headache)	SYMPTOMS	AURA (20-30 mins before)
☐ Alcohol	☐ Excessive Thirst	☐ Distorted Vision	☐ Black Spots
☐ Artificial Sweetener	☐ Excessive Yawning	☐ Dizziness	☐ Flashing Lights
☐ Beans	☐ Face Sensitivity	☐ Irritability	☐ Lack of Vision
☐ Caffeine	☐ Irritability	☐ Light-headedness	☐ Numbness FACE ARM LEG
☐ Cheese	☐ Light Sensitivity	☐ Light Sensitivity	☐ Zig Zag Lines
☐ Chocolate	☐ Neck Tightness	☐ Malaise	☐
☐ Fermented Foods	☐ Unexplained Fatigue	☐ Nasal Congestion	☐
☐ MSG	☐ Visual Disturbances	☐ Nausea/Vomiting	**TRIGGER & SYMPTOM NOTES**
☐ Non Friendly Fruits	☐	☐ Sound Sensitivity	
☐ Nuts	☐	☐ Tender Scalp	
☐ Processed Meats	☐	☐	
☐	☐	☐	
☐	☐	☐	
☐	☐		

REMEDIES

(NATURAL)		(OTC- COUNTER MEDS)	(Rx - PREVENTIVE)	(Rx - RELIEF)	(SUPPLEMENTS)
☐ Acupuncture	☐ Ice Pack	☐ Excedrin	☐ Amitriptyline	☐ Naproxin	☐ B2
☐ Acupressure	☐ Massage	☐ Ibuprofen	☐ Atenolol	☐ Nurtec	☐ Butterbur
☐ Caffeine	☐ Relaxation	☐ Tylenol	☐ Gabapentin	☐ Sumatriptan	☐ Feverfew
☐ Dark Room	☐ Silence	☐	☐ Nurtriptyline	☐ Rizatriptan	☐ Magnesium
☐ Hot Compress	☐ Walk	☐	☐ Propranolol	☐ Ubrelvy	☐
☐ Hydration	☐	☐	☐ Topamax	☐	☐
☐	☐	☐	☐ Valproate	☐	☐
☐	☐	☐	☐	WITHIN 1 HR OF PAIN YES NO	PAIN RELIEF YES NO
☐	☐	☐	☐		

REMEDY NOTES

IMPACT ON DAILY ACTIVITIES

NONE | MILD | MODERATE | SEVERE

WWW.ONEMINUTEMIGRAINEDIARY.COM

One Minute MIGRAINE Diary

Date : ______________________

Start Time : ________________ End Time : ____________ Duration : ________

PAIN SCALE [1-10]	MENSTRUAL PERIOD	PAIN TYPE	WATER
1 2 3 4 5 6 7 8 9 10 MILD MODERATE SEVERE	YES NO Birth Control Pills YES NO	Stabbing Burning Pulsating Shocking Pressure Pounding SLEEP	MISSED MEALS YES NO

PAIN LOCATION	WEATHER	STRESS
FRONT BACK LEFT RIGHT TOP	TEMP °	YES NO
	LIGHTS YES NO / SOUNDS YES NO	SMELLS YES NO

FOODS CONSUMED (within last 24 hours)	PRODROME (1-2 hours before headache)	SYMPTOMS	AURA (20-30 mins before)
☐ Alcohol	☐ Excessive Thirst	☐ Distorted Vision	☐ Black Spots
☐ Artificial Sweetener	☐ Excessive Yawning	☐ Dizziness	☐ Flashing Lights
☐ Beans	☐ Face Sensitivity	☐ Irritability	☐ Lack of Vision
☐ Caffeine	☐ Irritability	☐ Light-headedness	☐ Numbness FACE ARM LEG
☐ Cheese	☐ Light Sensitivity	☐ Light Sensitivity	☐ Zig Zag Lines
☐ Chocolate	☐ Neck Tightness	☐ Malaise	☐
☐ Fermented Foods	☐ Unexplained Fatigue	☐ Nasal Congestion	☐
☐ MSG	☐ Visual Disturbances	☐ Nausea/Vomiting	TRIGGER & SYMPTOM NOTES
☐ Non Friendly Fruits	☐	☐ Sound Sensitivity	
☐ Nuts	☐	☐ Tender Scalp	
☐ Processed Meats	☐	☐	
☐	☐	☐	
☐	☐	☐	
☐			

REMEDIES

(NATURAL)		(OTC- COUNTER MEDS)	(Rx - PREVENTIVE)	(Rx - RELIEF)	(SUPPLEMENTS)
☐ Acupuncture	☐ Ice Pack	☐ Excedrin	☐ Amitriptyline	☐ Naproxin	☐ B2
☐ Acupressure	☐ Massage	☐ Ibuprofen	☐ Atenolol	☐ Nurtec	☐ Butterbur
☐ Caffeine	☐ Relaxation	☐ Tylenol	☐ Gabapentin	☐ Sumatriptan	☐ Feverfew
☐ Dark Room	☐ Silence	☐	☐ Nurtriptyline	☐ Rizatriptan	☐ Magnesium
☐ Hot Compress	☐ Walk	☐	☐ Propranolol	☐ Ubrelvy	☐
☐ Hydration	☐	☐	☐ Topamax	☐	☐
☐	☐	☐	☐ Valproate	☐	☐
☐	☐	☐	☐	WITHIN 1 HR OF PAIN YES NO	PAIN RELIEF YES NO
☐	☐	☐	☐		

REMEDY NOTES

IMPACT ON DAILY ACTIVITIES

NONE | MILD | MODERATE | SEVERE

WWW.ONEMINUTEMIGRAINEDIARY.COM

One Minute MIGRAINE Diary

Date : ______________________

Start Time : ______________ End Time : ____________ Duration : ________

PAIN SCALE [1-10]

1 2 3 4 5 6 7 8 9 10

MILD MODERATE SEVERE

MENSTRUAL PERIOD

YES NO

Birth Control Pills

YES NO

PAIN TYPE

Stabbing Burning Pulsating Shocking Pressure Pounding

SLEEP

WATER

MISSED MEALS

YES NO

PAIN LOCATION

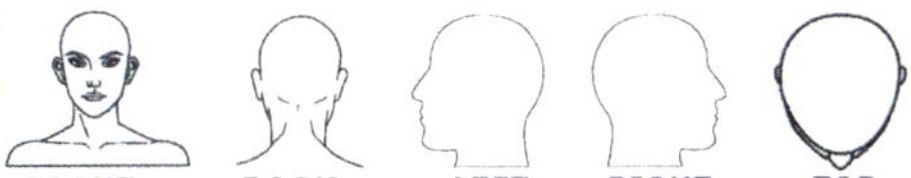

FRONT BACK LEFT RIGHT TOP

WEATHER

TEMP °

STRESS

YES NO

LIGHTS

YES NO

SOUNDS

YES NO

SMELLS

YES NO

FOODS CONSUMED (within last 24 hours)

- ☐ Alcohol
- ☐ Artificial Sweetener
- ☐ Beans
- ☐ Caffeine
- ☐ Cheese
- ☐ Chocolate
- ☐ Fermented Foods
- ☐ MSG
- ☐ Non Friendly Fruits
- ☐ Nuts
- ☐ Processed Meats
- ☐
- ☐
- ☐

PRODROME (1-2 hours before headache)

- ☐ Excessive Thirst
- ☐ Excessive Yawning
- ☐ Face Sensitivity
- ☐ Irritability
- ☐ Light Sensitivity
- ☐ Neck Tightness
- ☐ Unexplained Fatigue
- ☐ Visual Disturbances
- ☐
- ☐
- ☐
- ☐
- ☐

SYMPTOMS

- ☐ Distorted Vision
- ☐ Dizziness
- ☐ Irritability
- ☐ Light-headedness
- ☐ Light Sensitivity
- ☐ Malaise
- ☐ Nasal Congestion
- ☐ Nausea/Vomiting
- ☐ Sound Sensitivity
- ☐ Tender Scalp
- ☐
- ☐
- ☐

AURA (20-30 mins before)

- ☐ Black Spots
- ☐ Flashing Lights
- ☐ Lack of Vision
- ☐ Numbness FACE ARM LEG
- ☐ Zig Zag Lines
- ☐
- ☐

TRIGGER & SYMPTOM NOTES

REMEDIES

(NATURAL)

- ☐ Acupuncture
- ☐ Acupressure
- ☐ Caffeine
- ☐ Dark Room
- ☐ Hot Compress
- ☐ Hydration
- ☐
- ☐
- ☐
- ☐ Ice Pack
- ☐ Massage
- ☐ Relaxation
- ☐ Silence
- ☐ Walk
- ☐
- ☐
- ☐
- ☐

(OTC- COUNTER MEDS)

- ☐ Excedrin
- ☐ Ibuprofen
- ☐ Tylenol
- ☐
- ☐
- ☐
- ☐
- ☐
- ☐
- ☐

(Rx - PREVENTIVE)

- ☐ Amitriptyline
- ☐ Atenolol
- ☐ Gabapentin
- ☐ Nurtriptyline
- ☐ Propranolol
- ☐ Topamax
- ☐ Valproate
- ☐
- ☐

(Rx - RELIEF)

- ☐ Naproxin
- ☐ Nurtec
- ☐ Sumatriptan
- ☐ Rizatriptan
- ☐ Ubrelvy
- ☐
- ☐

(SUPPLEMENTS)

- ☐ B2
- ☐ Butterbur
- ☐ Feverfew
- ☐ Magnesium
- ☐
- ☐
- ☐

WITHIN 1 HR OF PAIN YES NO PAIN RELIEF YES NO

REMEDY NOTES

IMPACT ON DAILY ACTIVITIES

NONE | MILD | MODERATE | SEVERE

WWW.ONEMINUTEMIGRAINEDIARY.COM

One Minute

MIGRAINE Diary

Date : ____________________

Start Time : ____________ End Time : ____________ Duration : ________

PAIN SCALE [1-10]

1 2 3 4 5 6 7 8 9 10

MILD MODERATE SEVERE

MENSTRUAL PERIOD

YES NO

Birth Control Pills

YES NO

PAIN TYPE

Stabbing Burning Pulsating Shocking Pressure Pounding

SLEEP

WATER

MISSED MEALS

YES NO

PAIN LOCATION

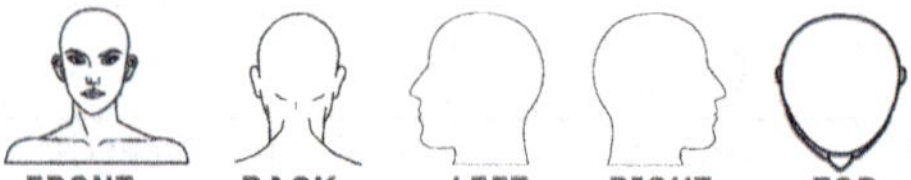

FRONT BACK LEFT RIGHT TOP

WEATHER

TEMP °

STRESS

YES NO

LIGHTS

YES NO

SOUNDS

YES NO

SMELLS

YES NO

FOODS CONSUMED (within last 24 hours)	PRODROME (1-2 hours before headache)	SYMPTOMS	AURA (20-30 mins before)
☐ Alcohol	☐ Excessive Thirst	☐ Distorted Vision	☐ Black Spots
☐ Artificial Sweetener	☐ Excessive Yawning	☐ Dizziness	☐ Flashing Lights
☐ Beans	☐ Face Sensitivity	☐ Irritability	☐ Lack of Vision
☐ Caffeine	☐ Irritability	☐ Light-headedness	☐ Numbness FACE ARM LEG
☐ Cheese	☐ Light Sensitivity	☐ Light Sensitivity	☐ Zig Zag Lines
☐ Chocolate	☐ Neck Tightness	☐ Malaise	☐
☐ Fermented Foods	☐ Unexplained Fatigue	☐ Nasal Congestion	☐
☐ MSG	☐ Visual Disturbances	☐ Nausea/Vomiting	**TRIGGER & SYMPTOM NOTES**
☐ Non Friendly Fruits	☐	☐ Sound Sensitivity	
☐ Nuts	☐	☐ Tender Scalp	
☐ Processed Meats	☐	☐	
☐	☐	☐	
☐	☐	☐	
☐	☐		

REMEDIES

(NATURAL)		(OTC- COUNTER MEDS)	(Rx - PREVENTIVE)	(Rx - RELIEF)	(SUPPLEMENTS)
☐ Acupuncture	☐ Ice Pack	☐ Excedrin	☐ Amitriptyline	☐ Naproxin	☐ B2
☐ Acupressure	☐ Massage	☐ Ibuprofen	☐ Atenolol	☐ Nurtec	☐ Butterbur
☐ Caffeine	☐ Relaxation	☐ Tylenol	☐ Gabapentin	☐ Sumatriptan	☐ Feverfew
☐ Dark Room	☐ Silence	☐	☐ Nurtriptyline	☐ Rizatriptan	☐ Magnesium
☐ Hot Compress	☐ Walk	☐	☐ Propranolol	☐ Ubrelvy	☐
☐ Hydration	☐	☐	☐ Topamax	☐	☐
☐	☐	☐	☐ Valproate	☐	☐
☐	☐	☐	☐	WITHIN 1 HR OF PAIN YES NO	PAIN RELIEF YES NO
☐	☐	☐	☐		

REMEDY NOTES

IMPACT ON DAILY ACTIVITIES

NONE | MILD | MODERATE | SEVERE

WWW.ONEMINUTEMIGRAINEDIARY.COM

One Minute MIGRAINE Diary

Date : ____________________

Start Time : ____________ End Time : ____________ Duration : ________

PAIN SCALE [1-10]	MENSTRUAL PERIOD	PAIN TYPE	WATER
1 2 3 4 5 6 7 8 9 10 MILD MODERATE SEVERE	YES NO Birth Control Pills YES NO	Stabbing Burning Pulsating Shocking Pressure Pounding SLEEP	MISSED MEALS YES NO
PAIN LOCATION FRONT BACK LEFT RIGHT TOP		WEATHER TEMP ° LIGHTS YES NO SOUNDS YES NO	STRESS YES NO SMELLS YES NO

FOODS CONSUMED (within last 24 hours)	PRODROME (1-2 hours before headache)	SYMPTOMS	AURA (20-30 mins before)
☐ Alcohol	☐ Excessive Thirst	☐ Distorted Vision	☐ Black Spots
☐ Artificial Sweetener	☐ Excessive Yawning	☐ Dizziness	☐ Flashing Lights
☐ Beans	☐ Face Sensitivity	☐ Irritability	☐ Lack of Vision
☐ Caffeine	☐ Irritability	☐ Light-headedness	☐ Numbness FACE ARM LEG
☐ Cheese	☐ Light Sensitivity	☐ Light Sensitivity	☐ Zig Zag Lines
☐ Chocolate	☐ Neck Tightness	☐ Malaise	☐
☐ Fermented Foods	☐ Unexplained Fatigue	☐ Nasal Congestion	☐
☐ MSG	☐ Visual Disturbances	☐ Nausea/Vomiting	TRIGGER & SYMPTOM NOTES
☐ Non Friendly Fruits	☐	☐ Sound Sensitivity	
☐ Nuts	☐	☐ Tender Scalp	
☐ Processed Meats	☐	☐	
☐	☐	☐	
☐	☐	☐	
☐			

REMEDIES

(NATURAL)		(OTC- COUNTER MEDS)	(Rx - PREVENTIVE)	(Rx - RELIEF)	(SUPPLEMENTS)
☐ Acupuncture	☐ Ice Pack	☐ Excedrin	☐ Amitriptyline	☐ Naproxin	☐ B2
☐ Acupressure	☐ Massage	☐ Ibuprofen	☐ Atenolol	☐ Nurtec	☐ Butterbur
☐ Caffeine	☐ Relaxation	☐ Tylenol	☐ Gabapentin	☐ Sumatriptan	☐ Feverfew
☐ Dark Room	☐ Silence	☐	☐ Nurtriptyline	☐ Rizatriptan	☐ Magnesium
☐ Hot Compress	☐ Walk	☐	☐ Propranolol	☐ Ubrelvy	☐
☐ Hydration	☐	☐	☐ Topamax	☐	☐
☐	☐	☐	☐ Valproate	☐	☐
☐	☐	☐	☐	WITHIN 1 HR OF PAIN YES NO	PAIN RELIEF YES NO
☐	☐	☐	☐		

REMEDY NOTES

IMPACT ON DAILY ACTIVITIES

NONE | MILD | MODERATE | SEVERE

WWW.ONEMINUTEMIGRAINEDIARY.COM

One Minute MIGRAINE Diary

Date : ______________________

Start Time : ________________ End Time : ____________ Duration : _______

PAIN SCALE [1-10]	MENSTRUAL PERIOD	PAIN TYPE	WATER
1 2 3 4 5 6 7 8 9 10 MILD MODERATE SEVERE	YES NO Birth Control Pills YES NO	Stabbing Burning Pulsating Shocking Pressure Pounding SLEEP	MISSED MEALS YES NO
PAIN LOCATION FRONT BACK LEFT RIGHT TOP		WEATHER TEMP	STRESS YES NO
		LIGHTS YES NO / SOUNDS YES NO	SMELLS YES NO

FOODS CONSUMED (within last 24 hours)	PRODROME (1-2 hours before headache)	SYMPTOMS	AURA (20-30 mins before)
☐ Alcohol	☐ Excessive Thirst	☐ Distorted Vision	☐ Black Spots
☐ Artificial Sweetener	☐ Excessive Yawning	☐ Dizziness	☐ Flashing Lights
☐ Beans	☐ Face Sensitivity	☐ Irritability	☐ Lack of Vision
☐ Caffeine	☐ Irritability	☐ Light-headedness	☐ Numbness FACE ARM LEG
☐ Cheese	☐ Light Sensitivity	☐ Light Sensitivity	☐ Zig Zag Lines
☐ Chocolate	☐ Neck Tightness	☐ Malaise	☐
☐ Fermented Foods	☐ Unexplained Fatigue	☐ Nasal Congestion	☐
☐ MSG	☐ Visual Disturbances	☐ Nausea/Vomiting	TRIGGER & SYMPTOM NOTES
☐ Non Friendly Fruits	☐	☐ Sound Sensitivity	
☐ Nuts	☐	☐ Tender Scalp	
☐ Processed Meats	☐	☐	
☐	☐	☐	
☐	☐	☐	
☐	☐		

REMEDIES

(NATURAL)		(OTC- COUNTER MEDS)	(Rx - PREVENTIVE)	(Rx - RELIEF)	(SUPPLEMENTS)
☐ Acupuncture	☐ Ice Pack	☐ Excedrin	☐ Amitriptyline	☐ Naproxin	☐ B2
☐ Acupressure	☐ Massage	☐ Ibuprofen	☐ Atenolol	☐ Nurtec	☐ Butterbur
☐ Caffeine	☐ Relaxation	☐ Tylenol	☐ Gabapentin	☐ Sumatriptan	☐ Feverfew
☐ Dark Room	☐ Silence	☐	☐ Nurtriptyline	☐ Rizatriptan	☐ Magnesium
☐ Hot Compress	☐ Walk	☐	☐ Propranolol	☐ Ubrelvy	☐
☐ Hydration	☐	☐	☐ Topamax	☐	☐
☐	☐	☐	☐ Valproate	☐	☐
☐	☐	☐	☐	WITHIN 1 HR OF PAIN YES NO	PAIN RELIEF YES NO
☐	☐	☐	☐		

REMEDY NOTES

IMPACT ON DAILY ACTIVITIES

NONE | MILD | MODERATE | SEVERE

WWW.ONEMINUTEMIGRAINEDIARY.COM

One Minute
MIGRAINE Diary

Date : ____________

Start Time : ____________ End Time : ____________ Duration : ____________

PAIN SCALE [1-10]

1 2 3 4 5 6 7 8 9 10

MILD MODERATE SEVERE

MENSTRUAL PERIOD

YES NO

Birth Control Pills

YES NO

PAIN TYPE

Stabbing Burning Pulsating Shocking Pressure Pounding

SLEEP

WATER

MISSED MEALS

YES NO

PAIN LOCATION

FRONT BACK LEFT RIGHT TOP

WEATHER

TEMP °

STRESS

YES NO

LIGHTS

YES NO

SOUNDS

YES NO

SMELLS

YES NO

FOODS CONSUMED (within last 24 hours)

- ☐ Alcohol
- ☐ Artificial Sweetener
- ☐ Beans
- ☐ Caffeine
- ☐ Cheese
- ☐ Chocolate
- ☐ Fermented Foods
- ☐ MSG
- ☐ Non Friendly Fruits
- ☐ Nuts
- ☐ Processed Meats
- ☐
- ☐
- ☐

PRODROME (1-2 hours before headache)

- ☐ Excessive Thirst
- ☐ Excessive Yawning
- ☐ Face Sensitivity
- ☐ Irritability
- ☐ Light Sensitivity
- ☐ Neck Tightness
- ☐ Unexplained Fatigue
- ☐ Visual Disturbances
- ☐
- ☐
- ☐
- ☐
- ☐

SYMPTOMS

- ☐ Distorted Vision
- ☐ Dizziness
- ☐ Irritability
- ☐ Light-headedness
- ☐ Light Sensitivity
- ☐ Malaise
- ☐ Nasal Congestion
- ☐ Nausea/Vomiting
- ☐ Sound Sensitivity
- ☐ Tender Scalp
- ☐
- ☐
- ☐

AURA (20-30 mins before)

- ☐ Black Spots
- ☐ Flashing Lights
- ☐ Lack of Vision
- ☐ Numbness FACE ARM LEG
- ☐ Zig Zag Lines
- ☐
- ☐

TRIGGER & SYMPTOM NOTES

REMEDIES

(NATURAL)

- ☐ Acupuncture
- ☐ Acupressure
- ☐ Caffeine
- ☐ Dark Room
- ☐ Hot Compress
- ☐ Hydration
- ☐
- ☐
- ☐
- ☐ Ice Pack
- ☐ Massage
- ☐ Relaxation
- ☐ Silence
- ☐ Walk
- ☐
- ☐
- ☐
- ☐

(OTC- COUNTER MEDS)

- ☐ Excedrin
- ☐ Ibuprofen
- ☐ Tylenol
- ☐
- ☐
- ☐
- ☐
- ☐
- ☐

(Rx - PREVENTIVE)

- ☐ Amitriptyline
- ☐ Atenolol
- ☐ Gabapentin
- ☐ Nurtriptyline
- ☐ Propranolol
- ☐ Topamax
- ☐ Valproate
- ☐
- ☐

(Rx - RELIEF)

- ☐ Naproxin
- ☐ Nurtec
- ☐ Sumatriptan
- ☐ Rizatriptan
- ☐ Ubrelvy
- ☐
- ☐

(SUPPLEMENTS)

- ☐ B2
- ☐ Butterbur
- ☐ Feverfew
- ☐ Magnesium
- ☐
- ☐
- ☐

WITHIN 1 HR OF PAIN YES NO PAIN RELIEF YES NO

REMEDY NOTES

IMPACT ON DAILY ACTIVITIES

NONE | MILD | MODERATE | SEVERE

WWW.ONEMINUTEMIGRAINEDIARY.COM

One Minute MIGRAINE Diary

Date : ____________________

Start Time : ______________ End Time : ______________ Duration : __________

PAIN SCALE [1-10] 1 2 3 4 5 6 7 8 9 10 MILD MODERATE SEVERE	**MENSTRUAL PERIOD** YES NO Birth Control Pills YES NO	**PAIN TYPE** Stabbing Burning Pulsating Shocking Pressure Pounding **SLEEP**	**WATER** **MISSED MEALS** YES NO
PAIN LOCATION FRONT BACK LEFT RIGHT TOP		**WEATHER** TEMP ° **LIGHTS** YES NO **SOUNDS** YES NO	**STRESS** YES NO **SMELLS** YES NO

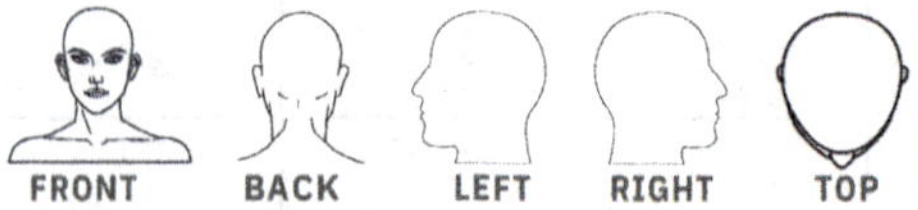

FOODS CONSUMED
(within last 24 hours)

- ☐ Alcohol
- ☐ Artificial Sweetener
- ☐ Beans
- ☐ Caffeine
- ☐ Cheese
- ☐ Chocolate
- ☐ Fermented Foods
- ☐ MSG
- ☐ Non Friendly Fruits
- ☐ Nuts
- ☐ Processed Meats
- ☐
- ☐
- ☐

PRODROME
(1-2 hours before headache)

- ☐ Excessive Thirst
- ☐ Excessive Yawning
- ☐ Face Sensitivity
- ☐ Irritability
- ☐ Light Sensitivity
- ☐ Neck Tightness
- ☐ Unexplained Fatigue
- ☐ Visual Disturbances
- ☐
- ☐
- ☐
- ☐
- ☐

SYMPTOMS

- ☐ Distorted Vision
- ☐ Dizziness
- ☐ Irritability
- ☐ Light-headedness
- ☐ Light Sensitivity
- ☐ Malaise
- ☐ Nasal Congestion
- ☐ Nausea/Vomiting
- ☐ Sound Sensitivity
- ☐ Tender Scalp
- ☐
- ☐
- ☐

AURA
(20-30 mins before)

- ☐ Black Spots
- ☐ Flashing Lights
- ☐ Lack of Vision
- ☐ Numbness FACE ARM LEG
- ☐ Zig Zag Lines
- ☐
- ☐

TRIGGER & SYMPTOM NOTES

REMEDIES

(NATURAL)

- ☐ Acupuncture
- ☐ Acupressure
- ☐ Caffeine
- ☐ Dark Room
- ☐ Hot Compress
- ☐ Hydration
- ☐
- ☐
- ☐
- ☐ Ice Pack
- ☐ Massage
- ☐ Relaxation
- ☐ Silence
- ☐ Walk
- ☐
- ☐
- ☐
- ☐

(OTC- COUNTER MEDS)

- ☐ Excedrin
- ☐ Ibuprofen
- ☐ Tylenol
- ☐
- ☐
- ☐
- ☐
- ☐
- ☐

(Rx - PREVENTIVE)

- ☐ Amitriptyline
- ☐ Atenolol
- ☐ Gabapentin
- ☐ Nurtriptyline
- ☐ Propranolol
- ☐ Topamax
- ☐ Valproate
- ☐
- ☐

(Rx - RELIEF)

- ☐ Naproxin
- ☐ Nurtec
- ☐ Sumatriptan
- ☐ Rizatriptan
- ☐ Ubrelvy
- ☐
- ☐

(SUPPLEMENTS)

- ☐ B2
- ☐ Butterbur
- ☐ Feverfew
- ☐ Magnesium
- ☐
- ☐
- ☐

WITHIN 1 HR OF PAIN YES NO PAIN RELIEF YES NO

REMEDY NOTES

IMPACT ON DAILY ACTIVITIES

NONE | MILD | MODERATE | SEVERE

WWW.ONEMINUTEMIGRAINEDIARY.COM

One Minute MIGRAINE Diary

Date : ______________________

Start Time : ______________ End Time : ____________ Duration : ________

PAIN SCALE [1-10]	MENSTRUAL PERIOD	PAIN TYPE	WATER
1 2 3 4 5 6 7 8 9 10 MILD MODERATE SEVERE	YES NO Birth Control Pills YES NO	Stabbing Burning Pulsating Shocking Pressure Pounding SLEEP	MISSED MEALS YES NO

PAIN LOCATION	WEATHER	STRESS
FRONT BACK LEFT RIGHT TOP	TEMP °	YES NO
	LIGHTS YES NO / SOUNDS YES NO	SMELLS YES NO

FOODS CONSUMED (within last 24 hours)	PRODROME (1-2 hours before headache)	SYMPTOMS	AURA (20-30 mins before)
☐ Alcohol	☐ Excessive Thirst	☐ Distorted Vision	☐ Black Spots
☐ Artificial Sweetener	☐ Excessive Yawning	☐ Dizziness	☐ Flashing Lights
☐ Beans	☐ Face Sensitivity	☐ Irritability	☐ Lack of Vision
☐ Caffeine	☐ Irritability	☐ Light-headedness	☐ Numbness FACE ARM LEG
☐ Cheese	☐ Light Sensitivity	☐ Light Sensitivity	☐ Zig Zag Lines
☐ Chocolate	☐ Neck Tightness	☐ Malaise	☐
☐ Fermented Foods	☐ Unexplained Fatigue	☐ Nasal Congestion	☐
☐ MSG	☐ Visual Disturbances	☐ Nausea/Vomiting	TRIGGER & SYMPTOM NOTES
☐ Non Friendly Fruits	☐	☐ Sound Sensitivity	
☐ Nuts	☐	☐ Tender Scalp	
☐ Processed Meats	☐	☐	
☐	☐	☐	
☐	☐	☐	
☐	☐		

REMEDIES

(NATURAL)		(OTC- COUNTER MEDS)	(Rx - PREVENTIVE)	(Rx - RELIEF)	(SUPPLEMENTS)
☐ Acupuncture	☐ Ice Pack	☐ Excedrin	☐ Amitriptyline	☐ Naproxin	☐ B2
☐ Acupressure	☐ Massage	☐ Ibuprofen	☐ Atenolol	☐ Nurtec	☐ Butterbur
☐ Caffeine	☐ Relaxation	☐ Tylenol	☐ Gabapentin	☐ Sumatriptan	☐ Feverfew
☐ Dark Room	☐ Silence	☐	☐ Nurtriptyline	☐ Rizatriptan	☐ Magnesium
☐ Hot Compress	☐ Walk	☐	☐ Propranolol	☐ Ubrelvy	☐
☐ Hydration	☐	☐	☐ Topamax	☐	☐
☐	☐	☐	☐ Valproate	☐	☐
☐	☐	☐	☐	WITHIN 1 HR OF PAIN YES NO	PAIN RELIEF YES NO
☐	☐	☐	☐		

REMEDY NOTES

IMPACT ON DAILY ACTIVITIES

NONE | MILD | MODERATE | SEVERE

WWW.ONEMINUTEMIGRAINEDIARY.COM

One Minute MIGRAINE Diary

Date : ____________________

Start Time : ____________ End Time : ____________ Duration : ________

PAIN SCALE [1-10]	MENSTRUAL PERIOD	PAIN TYPE	WATER
1 2 3 4 5 6 7 8 9 10 MILD MODERATE SEVERE	YES NO Birth Control Pills YES NO	Stabbing Burning Pulsating Shocking Pressure Pounding SLEEP	MISSED MEALS YES NO

PAIN LOCATION	WEATHER	STRESS
FRONT BACK LEFT RIGHT TOP	° TEMP	YES NO
	LIGHTS YES NO / SOUNDS YES NO	SMELLS YES NO

FOODS CONSUMED (within last 24 hours)	PRODROME (1-2 hours before headache)	SYMPTOMS	AURA (20-30 mins before)
☐ Alcohol	☐ Excessive Thirst	☐ Distorted Vision	☐ Black Spots
☐ Artificial Sweetener	☐ Excessive Yawning	☐ Dizziness	☐ Flashing Lights
☐ Beans	☐ Face Sensitivity	☐ Irritability	☐ Lack of Vision
☐ Caffeine	☐ Irritability	☐ Light-headedness	☐ Numbness FACE ARM LEG
☐ Cheese	☐ Light Sensitivity	☐ Light Sensitivity	☐ Zig Zag Lines
☐ Chocolate	☐ Neck Tightness	☐ Malaise	☐
☐ Fermented Foods	☐ Unexplained Fatigue	☐ Nasal Congestion	☐
☐ MSG	☐ Visual Disturbances	☐ Nausea/Vomiting	TRIGGER & SYMPTOM NOTES
☐ Non Friendly Fruits	☐	☐ Sound Sensitivity	
☐ Nuts	☐	☐ Tender Scalp	
☐ Processed Meats	☐	☐	
☐	☐	☐	
☐	☐	☐	
☐			

REMEDIES

(NATURAL)		(OTC- COUNTER MEDS)	(Rx - PREVENTIVE)	(Rx - RELIEF)	(SUPPLEMENTS)
☐ Acupuncture	☐ Ice Pack	☐ Excedrin	☐ Amitriptyline	☐ Naproxin	☐ B2
☐ Acupressure	☐ Massage	☐ Ibuprofen	☐ Atenolol	☐ Nurtec	☐ Butterbur
☐ Caffeine	☐ Relaxation	☐ Tylenol	☐ Gabapentin	☐ Sumatriptan	☐ Feverfew
☐ Dark Room	☐ Silence	☐	☐ Nurtriptyline	☐ Rizatriptan	☐ Magnesium
☐ Hot Compress	☐ Walk	☐	☐ Propranolol	☐ Ubrelvy	☐
☐ Hydration	☐	☐	☐ Topamax	☐	☐
☐	☐	☐	☐ Valproate	☐	☐
☐	☐	☐	☐	WITHIN 1 HR OF PAIN YES NO	PAIN RELIEF YES NO
☐	☐	☐	☐		

REMEDY NOTES

IMPACT ON DAILY ACTIVITIES

NONE | MILD | MODERATE | SEVERE

WWW.ONEMINUTEMIGRAINEDIARY.COM

One Minute MIGRAINE Diary

Date : ____________________

Start Time : ______________ End Time : ______________ Duration : __________

PAIN SCALE [1-10]

|-----|-----|-----|-----|-----|-----|-----|-----|-----|
1 2 3 4 5 6 7 8 9 10
MILD MODERATE SEVERE

MENSTRUAL PERIOD
YES NO
Birth Control Pills
YES NO

PAIN TYPE
Stabbing Burning Pulsating Shocking Pressure Pounding

SLEEP

WATER

MISSED MEALS
YES NO

PAIN LOCATION

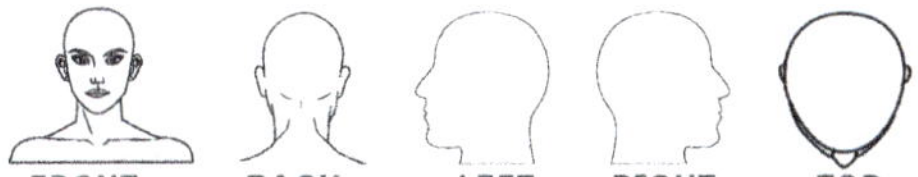

FRONT BACK LEFT RIGHT TOP

WEATHER
° TEMP

STRESS
YES NO

LIGHTS
YES NO

SOUNDS
YES NO

SMELLS
YES NO

FOODS CONSUMED (within last 24 hours)
- ☐ Alcohol
- ☐ Artificial Sweetener
- ☐ Beans
- ☐ Caffeine
- ☐ Cheese
- ☐ Chocolate
- ☐ Fermented Foods
- ☐ MSG
- ☐ Non Friendly Fruits
- ☐ Nuts
- ☐ Processed Meats
- ☐
- ☐
- ☐

PRODROME (1-2 hours before headache)
- ☐ Excessive Thirst
- ☐ Excessive Yawning
- ☐ Face Sensitivity
- ☐ Irritability
- ☐ Light Sensitivity
- ☐ Neck Tightness
- ☐ Unexplained Fatigue
- ☐ Visual Disturbances
- ☐
- ☐
- ☐
- ☐
- ☐

SYMPTOMS
- ☐ Distorted Vision
- ☐ Dizziness
- ☐ Irritability
- ☐ Light-headedness
- ☐ Light Sensitivity
- ☐ Malaise
- ☐ Nasal Congestion
- ☐ Nausea/Vomiting
- ☐ Sound Sensitivity
- ☐ Tender Scalp
- ☐
- ☐
- ☐

AURA (20-30 mins before)
- ☐ Black Spots
- ☐ Flashing Lights
- ☐ Lack of Vision
- ☐ Numbness FACE ARM LEG
- ☐ Zig Zag Lines
- ☐
- ☐

TRIGGER & SYMPTOM NOTES

REMEDIES

(NATURAL)
- ☐ Acupuncture
- ☐ Acupressure
- ☐ Caffeine
- ☐ Dark Room
- ☐ Hot Compress
- ☐ Hydration
- ☐
- ☐
- ☐
- ☐ Ice Pack
- ☐ Massage
- ☐ Relaxation
- ☐ Silence
- ☐ Walk
- ☐
- ☐
- ☐
- ☐

(OTC- COUNTER MEDS)
- ☐ Excedrin
- ☐ Ibuprofen
- ☐ Tylenol
- ☐
- ☐
- ☐
- ☐
- ☐
- ☐

(Rx - PREVENTIVE)
- ☐ Amitriptyline
- ☐ Atenolol
- ☐ Gabapentin
- ☐ Nurtriptyline
- ☐ Propranolol
- ☐ Topamax
- ☐ Valproate
- ☐
- ☐

(Rx - RELIEF)
- ☐ Naproxin
- ☐ Nurtec
- ☐ Sumatriptan
- ☐ Rizatriptan
- ☐ Ubrelvy
- ☐
- ☐

(SUPPLEMENTS)
- ☐ B2
- ☐ Butterbur
- ☐ Feverfew
- ☐ Magnesium
- ☐
- ☐
- ☐

WITHIN 1 HR OF PAIN YES NO PAIN RELIEF YES NO

REMEDY NOTES

IMPACT ON DAILY ACTIVITIES
NONE | MILD | MODERATE | SEVERE

WWW.ONEMINUTEMIGRAINEDIARY.COM

One Minute MIGRAINE Diary

Date : ____________________

Start Time : ______________ End Time : ______________ Duration : ________

PAIN SCALE [1-10]

1 2 3 4 5 6 7 8 9 10

MILD MODERATE SEVERE

MENSTRUAL PERIOD

YES NO

Birth Control Pills

YES NO

PAIN TYPE

Stabbing Burning Pulsating Shocking Pressure Pounding

SLEEP

WATER

MISSED MEALS

YES NO

PAIN LOCATION

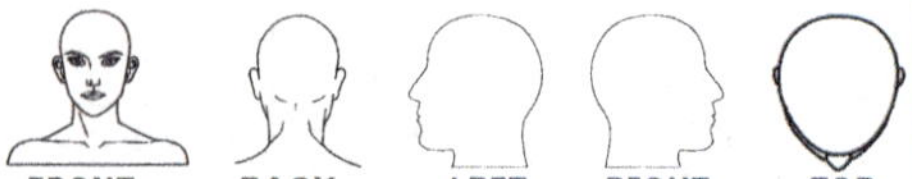

FRONT BACK LEFT RIGHT TOP

WEATHER

° TEMP

STRESS

YES NO

LIGHTS

YES NO

SOUNDS

YES NO

SMELLS

YES NO

FOODS CONSUMED (within last 24 hours)	PRODROME (1-2 hours before headache)	SYMPTOMS	AURA (20-30 mins before)
☐ Alcohol	☐ Excessive Thirst	☐ Distorted Vision	☐ Black Spots
☐ Artificial Sweetener	☐ Excessive Yawning	☐ Dizziness	☐ Flashing Lights
☐ Beans	☐ Face Sensitivity	☐ Irritability	☐ Lack of Vision
☐ Caffeine	☐ Irritability	☐ Light-headedness	☐ Numbness FACE ARM LEG
☐ Cheese	☐ Light Sensitivity	☐ Light Sensitivity	☐ Zig Zag Lines
☐ Chocolate	☐ Neck Tightness	☐ Malaise	☐
☐ Fermented Foods	☐ Unexplained Fatigue	☐ Nasal Congestion	☐
☐ MSG	☐ Visual Disturbances	☐ Nausea/Vomiting	**TRIGGER & SYMPTOM NOTES**
☐ Non Friendly Fruits	☐	☐ Sound Sensitivity	
☐ Nuts	☐	☐ Tender Scalp	
☐ Processed Meats	☐	☐	
☐	☐	☐	
☐	☐	☐	
☐	☐		

REMEDIES

(NATURAL)		(OTC- COUNTER MEDS)	(Rx - PREVENTIVE)	(Rx - RELIEF)	(SUPPLEMENTS)
☐ Acupuncture	☐ Ice Pack	☐ Excedrin	☐ Amitriptyline	☐ Naproxin	☐ B2
☐ Acupressure	☐ Massage	☐ Ibuprofen	☐ Atenolol	☐ Nurtec	☐ Butterbur
☐ Caffeine	☐ Relaxation	☐ Tylenol	☐ Gabapentin	☐ Sumatriptan	☐ Feverfew
☐ Dark Room	☐ Silence	☐	☐ Nurtriptyline	☐ Rizatriptan	☐ Magnesium
☐ Hot Compress	☐ Walk	☐	☐ Propranolol	☐ Ubrelvy	☐
☐ Hydration	☐	☐	☐ Topamax	☐	☐
☐	☐	☐	☐ Valproate	☐	☐
☐	☐	☐	☐	WITHIN 1 HR OF PAIN YES NO	PAIN RELIEF YES NO
☐	☐	☐	☐		

REMEDY NOTES

IMPACT ON DAILY ACTIVITIES

NONE | MILD | MODERATE | SEVERE

WWW.ONEMINUTEMIGRAINEDIARY.COM

One Minute MIGRAINE Diary

Date : ____________

Start Time : ____________ End Time : ____________ Duration : ________

PAIN SCALE [1-10]	MENSTRUAL PERIOD	PAIN TYPE	WATER
1 2 3 4 5 6 7 8 9 10 MILD MODERATE SEVERE	YES NO Birth Control Pills YES NO	Stabbing Burning Pulsating Shocking Pressure Pounding SLEEP	MISSED MEALS YES NO

PAIN LOCATION	WEATHER	STRESS
FRONT BACK LEFT RIGHT TOP	° TEMP	YES NO
	LIGHTS YES NO / SOUNDS YES NO	SMELLS YES NO

FOODS CONSUMED (within last 24 hours)	PRODROME (1-2 hours before headache)	SYMPTOMS	AURA (20-30 mins before)
☐ Alcohol	☐ Excessive Thirst	☐ Distorted Vision	☐ Black Spots
☐ Artificial Sweetener	☐ Excessive Yawning	☐ Dizziness	☐ Flashing Lights
☐ Beans	☐ Face Sensitivity	☐ Irritability	☐ Lack of Vision
☐ Caffeine	☐ Irritability	☐ Light-headedness	☐ Numbness FACE ARM LEG
☐ Cheese	☐ Light Sensitivity	☐ Light Sensitivity	☐ Zig Zag Lines
☐ Chocolate	☐ Neck Tightness	☐ Malaise	☐
☐ Fermented Foods	☐ Unexplained Fatigue	☐ Nasal Congestion	☐
☐ MSG	☐ Visual Disturbances	☐ Nausea/Vomiting	TRIGGER & SYMPTOM NOTES
☐ Non Friendly Fruits	☐	☐ Sound Sensitivity	
☐ Nuts	☐	☐ Tender Scalp	
☐ Processed Meats	☐	☐	
☐	☐	☐	
☐	☐	☐	
☐			

REMEDIES

(NATURAL)		(OTC- COUNTER MEDS)	(Rx - PREVENTIVE)	(Rx - RELIEF)	(SUPPLEMENTS)
☐ Acupuncture	☐ Ice Pack	☐ Excedrin	☐ Amitriptyline	☐ Naproxin	☐ B2
☐ Acupressure	☐ Massage	☐ Ibuprofen	☐ Atenolol	☐ Nurtec	☐ Butterbur
☐ Caffeine	☐ Relaxation	☐ Tylenol	☐ Gabapentin	☐ Sumatriptan	☐ Feverfew
☐ Dark Room	☐ Silence	☐	☐ Nurtriptyline	☐ Rizatriptan	☐ Magnesium
☐ Hot Compress	☐ Walk	☐	☐ Propranolol	☐ Ubrelvy	☐
☐ Hydration	☐	☐	☐ Topamax	☐	☐
☐	☐	☐	☐ Valproate	☐	☐
☐	☐	☐	☐	WITHIN 1 HR OF PAIN YES NO	PAIN RELIEF YES NO
☐	☐	☐	☐		

REMEDY NOTES

IMPACT ON DAILY ACTIVITIES

NONE | MILD | MODERATE | SEVERE

WWW.ONEMINUTEMIGRAINEDIARY.COM

One Minute
MIGRAINE Diary

Date : ______________________

Start Time : ______________ End Time : ____________ Duration : ________

PAIN SCALE [1-10]	MENSTRUAL PERIOD	PAIN TYPE	WATER
1 2 3 4 5 6 7 8 9 10 MILD MODERATE SEVERE	YES NO Birth Control Pills YES NO	Stabbing Burning Pulsating Shocking Pressure Pounding SLEEP	MISSED MEALS YES NO

PAIN LOCATION

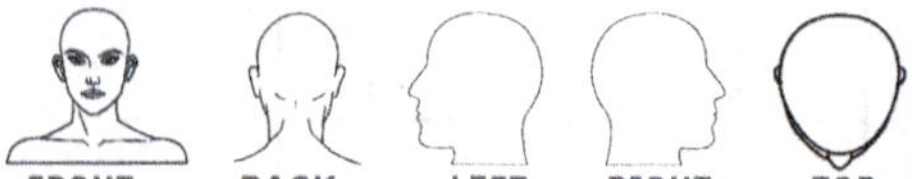

FRONT BACK LEFT RIGHT TOP

WEATHER

° TEMP

LIGHTS	SOUNDS	STRESS	SMELLS
YES NO	YES NO	YES NO	YES NO

FOODS CONSUMED (within last 24 hours)	PRODROME (1-2 hours before headache)	SYMPTOMS	AURA (20-30 mins before)
☐ Alcohol	☐ Excessive Thirst	☐ Distorted Vision	☐ Black Spots
☐ Artificial Sweetener	☐ Excessive Yawning	☐ Dizziness	☐ Flashing Lights
☐ Beans	☐ Face Sensitivity	☐ Irritability	☐ Lack of Vision
☐ Caffeine	☐ Irritability	☐ Light-headedness	☐ Numbness FACE ARM LEG
☐ Cheese	☐ Light Sensitivity	☐ Light Sensitivity	☐ Zig Zag Lines
☐ Chocolate	☐ Neck Tightness	☐ Malaise	☐
☐ Fermented Foods	☐ Unexplained Fatigue	☐ Nasal Congestion	☐
☐ MSG	☐ Visual Disturbances	☐ Nausea/Vomiting	TRIGGER & SYMPTOM NOTES
☐ Non Friendly Fruits	☐	☐ Sound Sensitivity	
☐ Nuts	☐	☐ Tender Scalp	
☐ Processed Meats	☐	☐	
☐	☐	☐	
☐	☐	☐	
☐	☐		

REMEDIES

(NATURAL)		(OTC- COUNTER MEDS)	(Rx - PREVENTIVE)	(Rx - RELIEF)	(SUPPLEMENTS)
☐ Acupuncture	☐ Ice Pack	☐ Excedrin	☐ Amitriptyline	☐ Naproxin	☐ B2
☐ Acupressure	☐ Massage	☐ Ibuprofen	☐ Atenolol	☐ Nurtec	☐ Butterbur
☐ Caffeine	☐ Relaxation	☐ Tylenol	☐ Gabapentin	☐ Sumatriptan	☐ Feverfew
☐ Dark Room	☐ Silence	☐	☐ Nurtriptyline	☐ Rizatriptan	☐ Magnesium
☐ Hot Compress	☐ Walk	☐	☐ Propranolol	☐ Ubrelvy	☐
☐ Hydration	☐	☐	☐ Topamax	☐	☐
☐	☐	☐	☐ Valproate	☐	☐
☐	☐	☐	☐	WITHIN 1 HR OF PAIN YES NO	PAIN RELIEF YES NO
☐	☐	☐	☐		

REMEDY NOTES

IMPACT ON DAILY ACTIVITIES

NONE | MILD | MODERATE | SEVERE

WWW.ONEMINUTEMIGRAINEDIARY.COM

One Minute MIGRAINE Diary

Date : ____________________

Start Time : ______________ End Time : ____________ Duration : ________

PAIN SCALE [1-10]

1 2 3 4 5 6 7 8 9 10

MILD MODERATE SEVERE

MENSTRUAL PERIOD

YES NO

Birth Control Pills

YES NO

PAIN TYPE

Stabbing Burning Pulsating Shocking Pressure Pounding

SLEEP

WATER

MISSED MEALS

YES NO

PAIN LOCATION

FRONT BACK LEFT RIGHT TOP

WEATHER

TEMP °

STRESS

YES NO

LIGHTS

YES NO

SOUNDS

YES NO

SMELLS

YES NO

FOODS CONSUMED (within last 24 hours)

- ☐ Alcohol
- ☐ Artificial Sweetener
- ☐ Beans
- ☐ Caffeine
- ☐ Cheese
- ☐ Chocolate
- ☐ Fermented Foods
- ☐ MSG
- ☐ Non Friendly Fruits
- ☐ Nuts
- ☐ Processed Meats
- ☐
- ☐
- ☐

PRODROME (1-2 hours before headache)

- ☐ Excessive Thirst
- ☐ Excessive Yawning
- ☐ Face Sensitivity
- ☐ Irritability
- ☐ Light Sensitivity
- ☐ Neck Tightness
- ☐ Unexplained Fatigue
- ☐ Visual Disturbances
- ☐
- ☐
- ☐
- ☐
- ☐

SYMPTOMS

- ☐ Distorted Vision
- ☐ Dizziness
- ☐ Irritability
- ☐ Light-headedness
- ☐ Light Sensitivity
- ☐ Malaise
- ☐ Nasal Congestion
- ☐ Nausea/Vomiting
- ☐ Sound Sensitivity
- ☐ Tender Scalp
- ☐
- ☐
- ☐

AURA (20-30 mins before)

- ☐ Black Spots
- ☐ Flashing Lights
- ☐ Lack of Vision
- ☐ Numbness FACE ARM LEG
- ☐ Zig Zag Lines
- ☐
- ☐

TRIGGER & SYMPTOM NOTES

REMEDIES

(NATURAL)

- ☐ Acupuncture
- ☐ Acupressure
- ☐ Caffeine
- ☐ Dark Room
- ☐ Hot Compress
- ☐ Hydration
- ☐
- ☐
- ☐
- ☐ Ice Pack
- ☐ Massage
- ☐ Relaxation
- ☐ Silence
- ☐ Walk
- ☐
- ☐
- ☐
- ☐

(OTC- COUNTER MEDS)

- ☐ Excedrin
- ☐ Ibuprofen
- ☐ Tylenol
- ☐
- ☐
- ☐
- ☐
- ☐
- ☐

(Rx - PREVENTIVE)

- ☐ Amitriptyline
- ☐ Atenolol
- ☐ Gabapentin
- ☐ Nurtriptyline
- ☐ Propranolol
- ☐ Topamax
- ☐ Valproate
- ☐
- ☐

(Rx - RELIEF)

- ☐ Naproxin
- ☐ Nurtec
- ☐ Sumatriptan
- ☐ Rizatriptan
- ☐ Ubrelvy
- ☐
- ☐

(SUPPLEMENTS)

- ☐ B2
- ☐ Butterbur
- ☐ Feverfew
- ☐ Magnesium
- ☐
- ☐
- ☐

WITHIN 1 HR OF PAIN YES NO

PAIN RELIEF YES NO

REMEDY NOTES

IMPACT ON DAILY ACTIVITIES

NONE | MILD | MODERATE | SEVERE

WWW.ONEMINUTEMIGRAINEDIARY.COM

One Minute MIGRAINE Diary

Date : ____________________

Start Time : ____________ End Time : ____________ Duration : ________

PAIN SCALE [1-10]	MENSTRUAL PERIOD	PAIN TYPE	WATER
1 2 3 4 5 6 7 8 9 10 MILD MODERATE SEVERE	YES NO Birth Control Pills YES NO	Stabbing Burning Pulsating Shocking Pressure Pounding SLEEP	MISSED MEALS YES NO

PAIN LOCATION	WEATHER	STRESS
FRONT BACK LEFT RIGHT TOP	TEMP °	YES NO
	LIGHTS YES NO SOUNDS YES NO	SMELLS YES NO

FOODS CONSUMED (within last 24 hours)

- ☐ Alcohol
- ☐ Artificial Sweetener
- ☐ Beans
- ☐ Caffeine
- ☐ Cheese
- ☐ Chocolate
- ☐ Fermented Foods
- ☐ MSG
- ☐ Non Friendly Fruits
- ☐ Nuts
- ☐ Processed Meats
- ☐
- ☐
- ☐

PRODROME (1-2 hours before headache)

- ☐ Excessive Thirst
- ☐ Excessive Yawning
- ☐ Face Sensitivity
- ☐ Irritability
- ☐ Light Sensitivity
- ☐ Neck Tightness
- ☐ Unexplained Fatigue
- ☐ Visual Disturbances
- ☐
- ☐
- ☐
- ☐
- ☐

SYMPTOMS

- ☐ Distorted Vision
- ☐ Dizziness
- ☐ Irritability
- ☐ Light-headedness
- ☐ Light Sensitivity
- ☐ Malaise
- ☐ Nasal Congestion
- ☐ Nausea/Vomiting
- ☐ Sound Sensitivity
- ☐ Tender Scalp
- ☐
- ☐
- ☐

AURA (20-30 mins before)

- ☐ Black Spots
- ☐ Flashing Lights
- ☐ Lack of Vision
- ☐ Numbness FACE ARM LEG
- ☐ Zig Zag Lines
- ☐
- ☐

TRIGGER & SYMPTOM NOTES

REMEDIES

(NATURAL)

- ☐ Acupuncture
- ☐ Acupressure
- ☐ Caffeine
- ☐ Dark Room
- ☐ Hot Compress
- ☐ Hydration
- ☐
- ☐
- ☐
- ☐ Ice Pack
- ☐ Massage
- ☐ Relaxation
- ☐ Silence
- ☐ Walk
- ☐
- ☐
- ☐
- ☐

(OTC- COUNTER MEDS)

- ☐ Excedrin
- ☐ Ibuprofen
- ☐ Tylenol
- ☐
- ☐
- ☐
- ☐
- ☐
- ☐

(Rx - PREVENTIVE)

- ☐ Amitriptyline
- ☐ Atenolol
- ☐ Gabapentin
- ☐ Nurtriptyline
- ☐ Propranolol
- ☐ Topamax
- ☐ Valproate
- ☐
- ☐

(Rx - RELIEF)

- ☐ Naproxin
- ☐ Nurtec
- ☐ Sumatriptan
- ☐ Rizatriptan
- ☐ Ubrelvy
- ☐
- ☐

(SUPPLEMENTS)

- ☐ B2
- ☐ Butterbur
- ☐ Feverfew
- ☐ Magnesium
- ☐
- ☐
- ☐

WITHIN 1 HR OF PAIN YES NO   PAIN RELIEF YES NO

REMEDY NOTES

IMPACT ON DAILY ACTIVITIES

NONE | MILD | MODERATE | SEVERE

WWW.ONEMINUTEMIGRAINEDIARY.COM

One Minute MIGRAINE Diary

Date : ____________________

Start Time : ____________________ End Time : ____________ Duration : ________

PAIN SCALE [1-10]	MENSTRUAL PERIOD	PAIN TYPE	WATER
1 2 3 4 5 6 7 8 9 10 MILD MODERATE SEVERE	YES NO Birth Control Pills YES NO	Stabbing Burning Pulsating Shocking Pressure Pounding **SLEEP**	**MISSED MEALS** YES NO

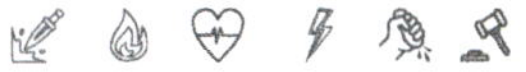

PAIN LOCATION

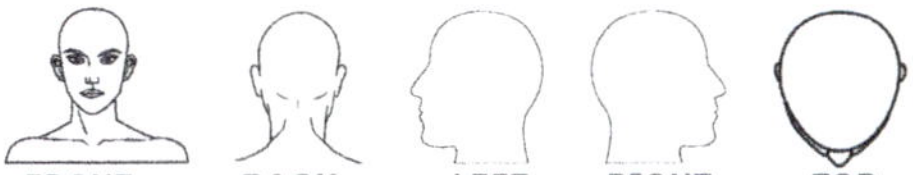

FRONT BACK LEFT RIGHT TOP

WEATHER

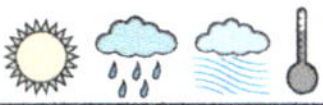

TEMP °

STRESS YES NO

LIGHTS YES NO

SOUNDS YES NO

SMELLS YES NO

FOODS CONSUMED (within last 24 hours)	PRODROME (1-2 hours before headache)	SYMPTOMS	AURA (20-30 mins before)
☐ Alcohol	☐ Excessive Thirst	☐ Distorted Vision	☐ Black Spots
☐ Artificial Sweetener	☐ Excessive Yawning	☐ Dizziness	☐ Flashing Lights
☐ Beans	☐ Face Sensitivity	☐ Irritability	☐ Lack of Vision
☐ Caffeine	☐ Irritability	☐ Light-headedness	☐ Numbness FACE ARM LEG
☐ Cheese	☐ Light Sensitivity	☐ Light Sensitivity	☐ Zig Zag Lines
☐ Chocolate	☐ Neck Tightness	☐ Malaise	☐
☐ Fermented Foods	☐ Unexplained Fatigue	☐ Nasal Congestion	☐
☐ MSG	☐ Visual Disturbances	☐ Nausea/Vomiting	**TRIGGER & SYMPTOM NOTES**
☐ Non Friendly Fruits	☐	☐ Sound Sensitivity	
☐ Nuts	☐	☐ Tender Scalp	
☐ Processed Meats	☐	☐	
☐	☐	☐	
☐	☐	☐	
☐			

REMEDIES

(NATURAL)		(OTC- COUNTER MEDS)	(Rx - PREVENTIVE)	(Rx - RELIEF)	(SUPPLEMENTS)
☐ Acupuncture	☐ Ice Pack	☐ Excedrin	☐ Amitriptyline	☐ Naproxin	☐ B2
☐ Acupressure	☐ Massage	☐ Ibuprofen	☐ Atenolol	☐ Nurtec	☐ Butterbur
☐ Caffeine	☐ Relaxation	☐ Tylenol	☐ Gabapentin	☐ Sumatriptan	☐ Feverfew
☐ Dark Room	☐ Silence	☐	☐ Nurtriptyline	☐ Rizatriptan	☐ Magnesium
☐ Hot Compress	☐ Walk	☐	☐ Propranolol	☐ Ubrelvy	☐
☐ Hydration	☐	☐	☐ Topamax	☐	☐
☐	☐	☐	☐ Valproate	☐	☐
☐	☐	☐	☐	WITHIN 1 HR OF PAIN YES NO	PAIN RELIEF YES NO
☐	☐	☐	☐		

REMEDY NOTES

IMPACT ON DAILY ACTIVITIES

NONE | MILD | MODERATE | SEVERE

WWW.ONEMINUTEMIGRAINEDIARY.COM

One Minute MIGRAINE Diary

Month

Migraine Tracking Prompts, Reflections and Assessments To Help You Track and Manage Your Migraines

WWW.ONEMINUTEMIGRAINEDIARY.COM

I am not my pain
My pain does not define me
I am not my pain
I am not defined by my pain
I am not my pain
I am strong, capable and confident

Book MEDIA Services

One Minute MIGRAINE Diary

Date : ______________________

Start Time : ______________ End Time : ______________ Duration : ________

PAIN SCALE [1-10]	MENSTRUAL PERIOD	PAIN TYPE	WATER
1 2 3 4 5 6 7 8 9 10 MILD MODERATE SEVERE	YES NO Birth Control Pills YES NO	Stabbing Burning Pulsating Shocking Pressure Pounding SLEEP	MISSED MEALS YES NO

PAIN LOCATION	WEATHER	STRESS
FRONT BACK LEFT RIGHT TOP	° TEMP	YES NO
	LIGHTS YES NO / SOUNDS YES NO	SMELLS YES NO

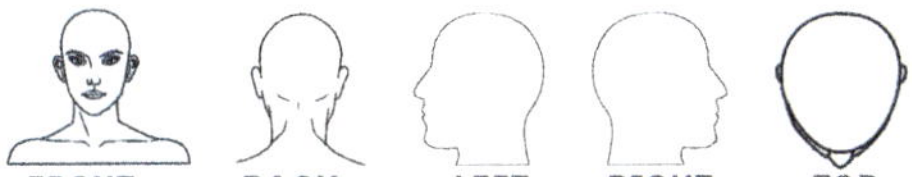

FOODS CONSUMED (within last 24 hours)	PRODROME (1-2 hours before headache)	SYMPTOMS	AURA (20-30 mins before)
☐ Alcohol	☐ Excessive Thirst	☐ Distorted Vision	☐ Black Spots
☐ Artificial Sweetener	☐ Excessive Yawning	☐ Dizziness	☐ Flashing Lights
☐ Beans	☐ Face Sensitivity	☐ Irritability	☐ Lack of Vision
☐ Caffeine	☐ Irritability	☐ Light-headedness	☐ Numbness FACE ARM LEG
☐ Cheese	☐ Light Sensitivity	☐ Light Sensitivity	☐ Zig Zag Lines
☐ Chocolate	☐ Neck Tightness	☐ Malaise	☐
☐ Fermented Foods	☐ Unexplained Fatigue	☐ Nasal Congestion	☐
☐ MSG	☐ Visual Disturbances	☐ Nausea/Vomiting	TRIGGER & SYMPTOM NOTES
☐ Non Friendly Fruits	☐	☐ Sound Sensitivity	
☐ Nuts	☐	☐ Tender Scalp	
☐ Processed Meats	☐	☐	
☐	☐	☐	
☐	☐	☐	
☐			

REMEDIES

(NATURAL)		(OTC- COUNTER MEDS)	(Rx - PREVENTIVE)	(Rx - RELIEF)	(SUPPLEMENTS)
☐ Acupuncture	☐ Ice Pack	☐ Excedrin	☐ Amitriptyline	☐ Naproxin	☐ B2
☐ Acupressure	☐ Massage	☐ Ibuprofen	☐ Atenolol	☐ Nurtec	☐ Butterbur
☐ Caffeine	☐ Relaxation	☐ Tylenol	☐ Gabapentin	☐ Sumatriptan	☐ Feverfew
☐ Dark Room	☐ Silence	☐	☐ Nurtriptyline	☐ Rizatriptan	☐ Magnesium
☐ Hot Compress	☐ Walk	☐	☐ Propranolol	☐ Ubrelvy	☐
☐ Hydration	☐	☐	☐ Topamax	☐	☐
☐	☐	☐	☐ Valproate	☐	☐
☐	☐	☐	☐	WITHIN 1 HR OF PAIN YES NO	PAIN RELIEF YES NO
☐	☐	☐	☐		

REMEDY NOTES

IMPACT ON DAILY ACTIVITIES

NONE | MILD | MODERATE | SEVERE

WWW.ONEMINUTEMIGRAINEDIARY.COM

One Minute MIGRAINE Diary

Date : ______________________

Start Time : ______________ End Time : ______________ Duration : ________

PAIN SCALE [1-10]

1 2 3 4 5 6 7 8 9 10

MILD MODERATE SEVERE

MENSTRUAL PERIOD

YES NO

Birth Control Pills

YES NO

PAIN TYPE

Stabbing Burning Pulsating Shocking Pressure Pounding

SLEEP

WATER

MISSED MEALS

YES NO

PAIN LOCATION

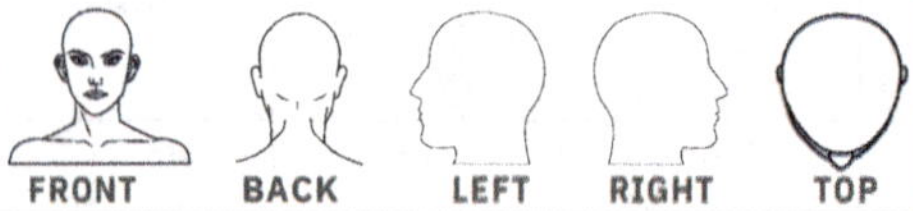

FRONT BACK LEFT RIGHT TOP

WEATHER

TEMP °

STRESS

YES NO

LIGHTS

YES NO

SOUNDS

YES NO

SMELLS

YES NO

FOODS CONSUMED (within last 24 hours)	PRODROME (1-2 hours before headache)	SYMPTOMS	AURA (20-30 mins before)
☐ Alcohol	☐ Excessive Thirst	☐ Distorted Vision	☐ Black Spots
☐ Artificial Sweetener	☐ Excessive Yawning	☐ Dizziness	☐ Flashing Lights
☐ Beans	☐ Face Sensitivity	☐ Irritability	☐ Lack of Vision
☐ Caffeine	☐ Irritability	☐ Light-headedness	☐ Numbness FACE ARM LEG
☐ Cheese	☐ Light Sensitivity	☐ Light Sensitivity	☐ Zig Zag Lines
☐ Chocolate	☐ Neck Tightness	☐ Malaise	☐
☐ Fermented Foods	☐ Unexplained Fatigue	☐ Nasal Congestion	☐
☐ MSG	☐ Visual Disturbances	☐ Nausea/Vomiting	**TRIGGER & SYMPTOM NOTES**
☐ Non Friendly Fruits	☐	☐ Sound Sensitivity	
☐ Nuts	☐	☐ Tender Scalp	
☐ Processed Meats	☐	☐	
☐	☐	☐	
☐	☐	☐	
☐			

REMEDIES

(NATURAL)		(OTC- COUNTER MEDS)	(Rx - PREVENTIVE)	(Rx - RELIEF)	(SUPPLEMENTS)
☐ Acupuncture	☐ Ice Pack	☐ Excedrin	☐ Amitriptyline	☐ Naproxin	☐ B2
☐ Acupressure	☐ Massage	☐ Ibuprofen	☐ Atenolol	☐ Nurtec	☐ Butterbur
☐ Caffeine	☐ Relaxation	☐ Tylenol	☐ Gabapentin	☐ Sumatriptan	☐ Feverfew
☐ Dark Room	☐ Silence	☐	☐ Nurtriptyline	☐ Rizatriptan	☐ Magnesium
☐ Hot Compress	☐ Walk	☐	☐ Propranolol	☐ Ubrelvy	☐
☐ Hydration	☐	☐	☐ Topamax	☐	☐
☐	☐	☐	☐ Valproate	☐	☐
☐	☐	☐	☐	WITHIN 1 HR OF PAIN YES NO	PAIN RELIEF YES NO
☐	☐	☐	☐		

REMEDY NOTES

IMPACT ON DAILY ACTIVITIES

NONE | MILD | MODERATE | SEVERE

WWW.ONEMINUTEMIGRAINEDIARY.COM

One Minute MIGRAINE Diary

Date : ______________________

Start Time : ______________ End Time : ______________ Duration : ________

PAIN SCALE [1-10]	MENSTRUAL PERIOD	PAIN TYPE	WATER
1 2 3 4 5 6 7 8 9 10 MILD MODERATE SEVERE	YES NO Birth Control Pills YES NO	Stabbing Burning Pulsating Shocking Pressure Pounding SLEEP	MISSED MEALS YES NO

PAIN LOCATION

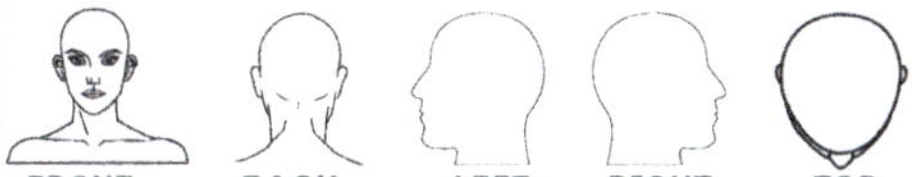

FRONT BACK LEFT RIGHT TOP

WEATHER	STRESS
TEMP °	YES NO
LIGHTS YES NO / SOUNDS YES NO	SMELLS YES NO

FOODS CONSUMED (within last 24 hours)	PRODROME (1-2 hours before headache)	SYMPTOMS	AURA (20-30 mins before)
☐ Alcohol	☐ Excessive Thirst	☐ Distorted Vision	☐ Black Spots
☐ Artificial Sweetener	☐ Excessive Yawning	☐ Dizziness	☐ Flashing Lights
☐ Beans	☐ Face Sensitivity	☐ Irritability	☐ Lack of Vision
☐ Caffeine	☐ Irritability	☐ Light-headedness	☐ Numbness FACE ARM LEG
☐ Cheese	☐ Light Sensitivity	☐ Light Sensitivity	☐ Zig Zag Lines
☐ Chocolate	☐ Neck Tightness	☐ Malaise	☐
☐ Fermented Foods	☐ Unexplained Fatigue	☐ Nasal Congestion	☐
☐ MSG	☐ Visual Disturbances	☐ Nausea/Vomiting	TRIGGER & SYMPTOM NOTES
☐ Non Friendly Fruits	☐	☐ Sound Sensitivity	
☐ Nuts	☐	☐ Tender Scalp	
☐ Processed Meats	☐	☐	
☐	☐	☐	
☐	☐	☐	
☐			

REMEDIES

(NATURAL)		(OTC- COUNTER MEDS)	(Rx - PREVENTIVE)	(Rx - RELIEF)	(SUPPLEMENTS)
☐ Acupuncture	☐ Ice Pack	☐ Excedrin	☐ Amitriptyline	☐ Naproxin	☐ B2
☐ Acupressure	☐ Massage	☐ Ibuprofen	☐ Atenolol	☐ Nurtec	☐ Butterbur
☐ Caffeine	☐ Relaxation	☐ Tylenol	☐ Gabapentin	☐ Sumatriptan	☐ Feverfew
☐ Dark Room	☐ Silence	☐	☐ Nurtriptyline	☐ Rizatriptan	☐ Magnesium
☐ Hot Compress	☐ Walk	☐	☐ Propranolol	☐ Ubrelvy	☐
☐ Hydration	☐	☐	☐ Topamax	☐	☐
☐	☐	☐	☐ Valproate	☐	☐
☐	☐	☐	☐	WITHIN 1 HR OF PAIN YES NO	PAIN RELIEF YES NO
☐	☐	☐	☐		

REMEDY NOTES

IMPACT ON DAILY ACTIVITIES

NONE | MILD | MODERATE | SEVERE

WWW.ONEMINUTEMIGRAINEDIARY.COM

One Minute
MIGRAINE Diary

Date : ______________________

Start Time : ______________ End Time : ____________ Duration : ________

PAIN SCALE [1-10]
1 2 3 4 5 6 7 8 9 10
MILD MODERATE SEVERE

MENSTRUAL PERIOD
YES NO
Birth Control Pills
YES NO

PAIN TYPE
Stabbing Burning Pulsating Shocking Pressure Pounding

SLEEP

WATER

MISSED MEALS
YES NO

PAIN LOCATION
FRONT BACK LEFT RIGHT TOP

WEATHER
TEMP °

STRESS
YES NO

LIGHTS
YES NO

SOUNDS
YES NO

SMELLS
YES NO

FOODS CONSUMED (within last 24 hours)
- ☐ Alcohol
- ☐ Artificial Sweetener
- ☐ Beans
- ☐ Caffeine
- ☐ Cheese
- ☐ Chocolate
- ☐ Fermented Foods
- ☐ MSG
- ☐ Non Friendly Fruits
- ☐ Nuts
- ☐ Processed Meats
- ☐
- ☐
- ☐

PRODROME (1-2 hours before headache)
- ☐ Excessive Thirst
- ☐ Excessive Yawning
- ☐ Face Sensitivity
- ☐ Irritability
- ☐ Light Sensitivity
- ☐ Neck Tightness
- ☐ Unexplained Fatigue
- ☐ Visual Disturbances
- ☐
- ☐
- ☐
- ☐
- ☐

SYMPTOMS
- ☐ Distorted Vision
- ☐ Dizziness
- ☐ Irritability
- ☐ Light-headedness
- ☐ Light Sensitivity
- ☐ Malaise
- ☐ Nasal Congestion
- ☐ Nausea/Vomiting
- ☐ Sound Sensitivity
- ☐ Tender Scalp
- ☐
- ☐
- ☐

AURA (20-30 mins before)
- ☐ Black Spots
- ☐ Flashing Lights
- ☐ Lack of Vision
- ☐ Numbness FACE ARM LEG
- ☐ Zig Zag Lines
- ☐
- ☐

TRIGGER & SYMPTOM NOTES

REMEDIES

(NATURAL)
- ☐ Acupuncture
- ☐ Acupressure
- ☐ Caffeine
- ☐ Dark Room
- ☐ Hot Compress
- ☐ Hydration
- ☐
- ☐
- ☐
- ☐ Ice Pack
- ☐ Massage
- ☐ Relaxation
- ☐ Silence
- ☐ Walk
- ☐
- ☐
- ☐
- ☐

(OTC- COUNTER MEDS)
- ☐ Excedrin
- ☐ Ibuprofen
- ☐ Tylenol
- ☐
- ☐
- ☐
- ☐
- ☐
- ☐

(Rx - PREVENTIVE)
- ☐ Amitriptyline
- ☐ Atenolol
- ☐ Gabapentin
- ☐ Nurtriptyline
- ☐ Propranolol
- ☐ Topamax
- ☐ Valproate
- ☐
- ☐

(Rx - RELIEF)
- ☐ Naproxin
- ☐ Nurtec
- ☐ Sumatriptan
- ☐ Rizatriptan
- ☐ Ubrelvy
- ☐
- ☐

(SUPPLEMENTS)
- ☐ B2
- ☐ Butterbur
- ☐ Feverfew
- ☐ Magnesium
- ☐
- ☐
- ☐

WITHIN 1 HR OF PAIN YES NO PAIN RELIEF YES NO

REMEDY NOTES

IMPACT ON DAILY ACTIVITIES
NONE | MILD | MODERATE | SEVERE

WWW.ONEMINUTEMIGRAINEDIARY.COM

One Minute MIGRAINE Diary

Date : ______________________

Start Time : ______________ End Time : ____________ Duration : ________

PAIN SCALE [1-10]	MENSTRUAL PERIOD	PAIN TYPE	WATER
1 2 3 4 5 6 7 8 9 10 MILD MODERATE SEVERE	YES NO Birth Control Pills YES NO	Stabbing Burning Pulsating Shocking Pressure Pounding SLEEP	MISSED MEALS YES NO

PAIN LOCATION	WEATHER	STRESS
FRONT BACK LEFT RIGHT TOP	TEMP °	YES NO
	LIGHTS YES NO / SOUNDS YES NO	SMELLS YES NO

FOODS CONSUMED (within last 24 hours)

- ☐ Alcohol
- ☐ Artificial Sweetener
- ☐ Beans
- ☐ Caffeine
- ☐ Cheese
- ☐ Chocolate
- ☐ Fermented Foods
- ☐ MSG
- ☐ Non Friendly Fruits
- ☐ Nuts
- ☐ Processed Meats
- ☐
- ☐
- ☐

PRODROME (1-2 hours before headache)

- ☐ Excessive Thirst
- ☐ Excessive Yawning
- ☐ Face Sensitivity
- ☐ Irritability
- ☐ Light Sensitivity
- ☐ Neck Tightness
- ☐ Unexplained Fatigue
- ☐ Visual Disturbances
- ☐
- ☐
- ☐
- ☐
- ☐

SYMPTOMS

- ☐ Distorted Vision
- ☐ Dizziness
- ☐ Irritability
- ☐ Light-headedness
- ☐ Light Sensitivity
- ☐ Malaise
- ☐ Nasal Congestion
- ☐ Nausea/Vomiting
- ☐ Sound Sensitivity
- ☐ Tender Scalp
- ☐
- ☐
- ☐

AURA (20-30 mins before)

- ☐ Black Spots
- ☐ Flashing Lights
- ☐ Lack of Vision
- ☐ Numbness FACE ARM LEG
- ☐ Zig Zag Lines
- ☐
- ☐

TRIGGER & SYMPTOM NOTES

REMEDIES

(NATURAL)

- ☐ Acupuncture
- ☐ Acupressure
- ☐ Caffeine
- ☐ Dark Room
- ☐ Hot Compress
- ☐ Hydration
- ☐
- ☐
- ☐
- ☐ Ice Pack
- ☐ Massage
- ☐ Relaxation
- ☐ Silence
- ☐ Walk
- ☐
- ☐
- ☐
- ☐

(OTC- COUNTER MEDS)

- ☐ Excedrin
- ☐ Ibuprofen
- ☐ Tylenol
- ☐
- ☐
- ☐
- ☐
- ☐
- ☐

(Rx - PREVENTIVE)

- ☐ Amitriptyline
- ☐ Atenolol
- ☐ Gabapentin
- ☐ Nurtriptyline
- ☐ Propranolol
- ☐ Topamax
- ☐ Valproate
- ☐
- ☐

(Rx - RELIEF)

- ☐ Naproxin
- ☐ Nurtec
- ☐ Sumatriptan
- ☐ Rizatriptan
- ☐ Ubrelvy
- ☐
- ☐

(SUPPLEMENTS)

- ☐ B2
- ☐ Butterbur
- ☐ Feverfew
- ☐ Magnesium
- ☐
- ☐
- ☐

WITHIN 1 HR OF PAIN YES NO PAIN RELIEF YES NO

REMEDY NOTES

IMPACT ON DAILY ACTIVITIES

NONE | MILD | MODERATE | SEVERE

WWW.ONEMINUTEMIGRAINEDIARY.COM

One Minute MIGRAINE Diary

Date : ____________________

Start Time : ______________ End Time : ______________ Duration : ________

PAIN SCALE [1-10]	MENSTRUAL PERIOD	PAIN TYPE	WATER
1 2 3 4 5 6 7 8 9 10 MILD MODERATE SEVERE	YES NO Birth Control Pills YES NO	Stabbing Burning Pulsating Shocking Pressure Pounding SLEEP	MISSED MEALS YES NO

PAIN LOCATION	WEATHER	STRESS
FRONT BACK LEFT RIGHT TOP	TEMP °	YES NO
	LIGHTS YES NO / SOUNDS YES NO	SMELLS YES NO

FOODS CONSUMED (within last 24 hours)	PRODROME (1-2 hours before headache)	SYMPTOMS	AURA (20-30 mins before)
☐ Alcohol	☐ Excessive Thirst	☐ Distorted Vision	☐ Black Spots
☐ Artificial Sweetener	☐ Excessive Yawning	☐ Dizziness	☐ Flashing Lights
☐ Beans	☐ Face Sensitivity	☐ Irritability	☐ Lack of Vision
☐ Caffeine	☐ Irritability	☐ Light-headedness	☐ Numbness FACE ARM LEG
☐ Cheese	☐ Light Sensitivity	☐ Light Sensitivity	☐ Zig Zag Lines
☐ Chocolate	☐ Neck Tightness	☐ Malaise	☐
☐ Fermented Foods	☐ Unexplained Fatigue	☐ Nasal Congestion	☐
☐ MSG	☐ Visual Disturbances	☐ Nausea/Vomiting	TRIGGER & SYMPTOM NOTES
☐ Non Friendly Fruits	☐	☐ Sound Sensitivity	
☐ Nuts	☐	☐ Tender Scalp	
☐ Processed Meats	☐	☐	
☐	☐	☐	
☐	☐	☐	
☐	☐		

REMEDIES

(NATURAL)		(OTC- COUNTER MEDS)	(Rx - PREVENTIVE)	(Rx - RELIEF)	(SUPPLEMENTS)
☐ Acupuncture	☐ Ice Pack	☐ Excedrin	☐ Amitriptyline	☐ Naproxin	☐ B2
☐ Acupressure	☐ Massage	☐ Ibuprofen	☐ Atenolol	☐ Nurtec	☐ Butterbur
☐ Caffeine	☐ Relaxation	☐ Tylenol	☐ Gabapentin	☐ Sumatriptan	☐ Feverfew
☐ Dark Room	☐ Silence	☐	☐ Nurtriptyline	☐ Rizatriptan	☐ Magnesium
☐ Hot Compress	☐ Walk	☐	☐ Propranolol	☐ Ubrelvy	☐
☐ Hydration	☐	☐	☐ Topamax	☐	☐
☐	☐	☐	☐ Valproate	☐	☐
☐	☐	☐	☐	WITHIN 1 HR OF PAIN YES NO	PAIN RELIEF YES NO
☐	☐	☐	☐		

REMEDY NOTES

IMPACT ON DAILY ACTIVITIES

NONE | MILD | MODERATE | SEVERE

WWW.ONEMINUTEMIGRAINEDIARY.COM

One Minute MIGRAINE Diary

Date : ______________________

Start Time : ______________ End Time : ____________ Duration : _______

PAIN SCALE [1-10]
1 2 3 4 5 6 7 8 9 10
MILD MODERATE SEVERE

MENSTRUAL PERIOD
YES NO
Birth Control Pills
YES NO

PAIN TYPE
Stabbing Burning Pulsating Shocking Pressure Pounding

SLEEP

WATER

MISSED MEALS
YES NO

PAIN LOCATION
FRONT BACK LEFT RIGHT TOP

WEATHER
TEMP °

STRESS
YES NO

LIGHTS
YES NO

SOUNDS
YES NO

SMELLS
YES NO

FOODS CONSUMED (within last 24 hours)
- ☐ Alcohol
- ☐ Artificial Sweetener
- ☐ Beans
- ☐ Caffeine
- ☐ Cheese
- ☐ Chocolate
- ☐ Fermented Foods
- ☐ MSG
- ☐ Non Friendly Fruits
- ☐ Nuts
- ☐ Processed Meats
- ☐
- ☐
- ☐

PRODROME (1-2 hours before headache)
- ☐ Excessive Thirst
- ☐ Excessive Yawning
- ☐ Face Sensitivity
- ☐ Irritability
- ☐ Light Sensitivity
- ☐ Neck Tightness
- ☐ Unexplained Fatigue
- ☐ Visual Disturbances
- ☐
- ☐
- ☐
- ☐
- ☐

SYMPTOMS
- ☐ Distorted Vision
- ☐ Dizziness
- ☐ Irritability
- ☐ Light-headedness
- ☐ Light Sensitivity
- ☐ Malaise
- ☐ Nasal Congestion
- ☐ Nausea/Vomiting
- ☐ Sound Sensitivity
- ☐ Tender Scalp
- ☐
- ☐
- ☐

AURA (20-30 mins before)
- ☐ Black Spots
- ☐ Flashing Lights
- ☐ Lack of Vision
- ☐ Numbness FACE ARM LEG
- ☐ Zig Zag Lines
- ☐
- ☐

TRIGGER & SYMPTOM NOTES

REMEDIES

(NATURAL)
- ☐ Acupuncture
- ☐ Acupressure
- ☐ Caffeine
- ☐ Dark Room
- ☐ Hot Compress
- ☐ Hydration
- ☐
- ☐
- ☐
- ☐ Ice Pack
- ☐ Massage
- ☐ Relaxation
- ☐ Silence
- ☐ Walk
- ☐
- ☐
- ☐
- ☐

(OTC- COUNTER MEDS)
- ☐ Excedrin
- ☐ Ibuprofen
- ☐ Tylenol
- ☐
- ☐
- ☐
- ☐
- ☐
- ☐

(Rx - PREVENTIVE)
- ☐ Amitriptyline
- ☐ Atenolol
- ☐ Gabapentin
- ☐ Nurtriptyline
- ☐ Propranolol
- ☐ Topamax
- ☐ Valproate
- ☐
- ☐

(Rx - RELIEF)
- ☐ Naproxin
- ☐ Nurtec
- ☐ Sumatriptan
- ☐ Rizatriptan
- ☐ Ubrelvy
- ☐
- ☐

(SUPPLEMENTS)
- ☐ B2
- ☐ Butterbur
- ☐ Feverfew
- ☐ Magnesium
- ☐
- ☐
- ☐

WITHIN 1 HR OF PAIN YES NO PAIN RELIEF YES NO

REMEDY NOTES

IMPACT ON DAILY ACTIVITIES
NONE | MILD | MODERATE | SEVERE

WWW.ONEMINUTEMIGRAINEDIARY.COM

One Minute MIGRAINE Diary

Date : ____________________

Start Time : ____________ End Time : ____________ Duration : ________

PAIN SCALE [1-10]	MENSTRUAL PERIOD	PAIN TYPE	WATER
1 2 3 4 5 6 7 8 9 10 MILD MODERATE SEVERE	YES NO Birth Control Pills YES NO	Stabbing Burning Pulsating Shocking Pressure Pounding SLEEP	MISSED MEALS YES NO

PAIN LOCATION	WEATHER	STRESS
FRONT BACK LEFT RIGHT TOP	TEMP °	YES NO
	LIGHTS YES NO · SOUNDS YES NO	SMELLS YES NO

FOODS CONSUMED (within last 24 hours)	PRODROME (1-2 hours before headache)	SYMPTOMS	AURA (20-30 mins before)
☐ Alcohol	☐ Excessive Thirst	☐ Distorted Vision	☐ Black Spots
☐ Artificial Sweetener	☐ Excessive Yawning	☐ Dizziness	☐ Flashing Lights
☐ Beans	☐ Face Sensitivity	☐ Irritability	☐ Lack of Vision
☐ Caffeine	☐ Irritability	☐ Light-headedness	☐ Numbness FACE ARM LEG
☐ Cheese	☐ Light Sensitivity	☐ Light Sensitivity	☐ Zig Zag Lines
☐ Chocolate	☐ Neck Tightness	☐ Malaise	☐
☐ Fermented Foods	☐ Unexplained Fatigue	☐ Nasal Congestion	☐
☐ MSG	☐ Visual Disturbances	☐ Nausea/Vomiting	TRIGGER & SYMPTOM NOTES
☐ Non Friendly Fruits	☐	☐ Sound Sensitivity	
☐ Nuts	☐	☐ Tender Scalp	
☐ Processed Meats	☐	☐	
☐	☐	☐	
☐	☐	☐	
☐	☐		

REMEDIES

(NATURAL)		(OTC- COUNTER MEDS)	(Rx - PREVENTIVE)	(Rx - RELIEF)	(SUPPLEMENTS)
☐ Acupuncture	☐ Ice Pack	☐ Excedrin	☐ Amitriptyline	☐ Naproxin	☐ B2
☐ Acupressure	☐ Massage	☐ Ibuprofen	☐ Atenolol	☐ Nurtec	☐ Butterbur
☐ Caffeine	☐ Relaxation	☐ Tylenol	☐ Gabapentin	☐ Sumatriptan	☐ Feverfew
☐ Dark Room	☐ Silence	☐	☐ Nurtriptyline	☐ Rizatriptan	☐ Magnesium
☐ Hot Compress	☐ Walk	☐	☐ Propranolol	☐ Ubrelvy	☐
☐ Hydration	☐	☐	☐ Topamax	☐	☐
☐	☐	☐	☐ Valproate	☐	☐
☐	☐	☐	☐	WITHIN 1 HR OF PAIN YES NO	PAIN RELIEF YES NO
☐	☐	☐	☐		

REMEDY NOTES

IMPACT ON DAILY ACTIVITIES

NONE | MILD | MODERATE | SEVERE

WWW.ONEMINUTEMIGRAINEDIARY.COM

One Minute MIGRAINE Diary

Date : ______________________

Start Time : ______________ End Time : ______________ Duration : ________

PAIN SCALE [1-10]

1 2 3 4 5 6 7 8 9 10

MILD MODERATE SEVERE

MENSTRUAL PERIOD

YES NO

Birth Control Pills

YES NO

PAIN TYPE

Stabbing Burning Pulsating Shocking Pressure Pounding

SLEEP

WATER

MISSED MEALS

YES NO

PAIN LOCATION

FRONT BACK LEFT RIGHT TOP

WEATHER

° TEMP

STRESS

YES NO

LIGHTS

YES NO

SOUNDS

YES NO

SMELLS

YES NO

FOODS CONSUMED (within last 24 hours)

- ☐ Alcohol
- ☐ Artificial Sweetener
- ☐ Beans
- ☐ Caffeine
- ☐ Cheese
- ☐ Chocolate
- ☐ Fermented Foods
- ☐ MSG
- ☐ Non Friendly Fruits
- ☐ Nuts
- ☐ Processed Meats
- ☐
- ☐
- ☐

PRODROME (1-2 hours before headache)

- ☐ Excessive Thirst
- ☐ Excessive Yawning
- ☐ Face Sensitivity
- ☐ Irritability
- ☐ Light Sensitivity
- ☐ Neck Tightness
- ☐ Unexplained Fatigue
- ☐ Visual Disturbances
- ☐
- ☐
- ☐
- ☐
- ☐

SYMPTOMS

- ☐ Distorted Vision
- ☐ Dizziness
- ☐ Irritability
- ☐ Light-headedness
- ☐ Light Sensitivity
- ☐ Malaise
- ☐ Nasal Congestion
- ☐ Nausea/Vomiting
- ☐ Sound Sensitivity
- ☐ Tender Scalp
- ☐
- ☐
- ☐

AURA (20-30 mins before)

- ☐ Black Spots
- ☐ Flashing Lights
- ☐ Lack of Vision
- ☐ Numbness FACE ARM LEG
- ☐ Zig Zag Lines
- ☐
- ☐

TRIGGER & SYMPTOM NOTES

REMEDIES

(NATURAL)

- ☐ Acupuncture
- ☐ Acupressure
- ☐ Caffeine
- ☐ Dark Room
- ☐ Hot Compress
- ☐ Hydration
- ☐
- ☐
- ☐
- ☐ Ice Pack
- ☐ Massage
- ☐ Relaxation
- ☐ Silence
- ☐ Walk
- ☐
- ☐
- ☐
- ☐

(OTC- COUNTER MEDS)

- ☐ Excedrin
- ☐ Ibuprofen
- ☐ Tylenol
- ☐
- ☐
- ☐
- ☐
- ☐
- ☐

(Rx - PREVENTIVE)

- ☐ Amitriptyline
- ☐ Atenolol
- ☐ Gabapentin
- ☐ Nurtriptyline
- ☐ Propranolol
- ☐ Topamax
- ☐ Valproate
- ☐
- ☐

(Rx - RELIEF)

- ☐ Naproxin
- ☐ Nurtec
- ☐ Sumatriptan
- ☐ Rizatriptan
- ☐ Ubrelvy
- ☐
- ☐

(SUPPLEMENTS)

- ☐ B2
- ☐ Butterbur
- ☐ Feverfew
- ☐ Magnesium
- ☐
- ☐
- ☐

WITHIN 1 HR OF PAIN YES NO PAIN RELIEF YES NO

REMEDY NOTES

IMPACT ON DAILY ACTIVITIES

NONE | MILD | MODERATE | SEVERE

One Minute MIGRAINE Diary

Date : ____________________

Start Time : ______________ End Time : ____________ Duration : ________

PAIN SCALE [1-10]	MENSTRUAL PERIOD	PAIN TYPE	WATER
1 2 3 4 5 6 7 8 9 10 MILD MODERATE SEVERE	YES NO Birth Control Pills YES NO	Stabbing Burning Pulsating Shocking Pressure Pounding **SLEEP**	**MISSED MEALS** YES NO

PAIN LOCATION

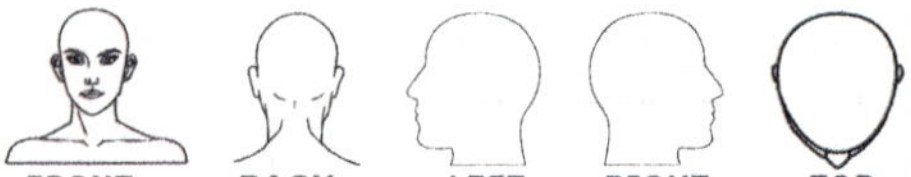

FRONT BACK LEFT RIGHT TOP

WEATHER

TEMP °

STRESS YES NO

LIGHTS YES NO **SOUNDS** YES NO **SMELLS** YES NO

FOODS CONSUMED (within last 24 hours)	PRODROME (1-2 hours before headache)	SYMPTOMS	AURA (20-30 mins before)
☐ Alcohol	☐ Excessive Thirst	☐ Distorted Vision	☐ Black Spots
☐ Artificial Sweetener	☐ Excessive Yawning	☐ Dizziness	☐ Flashing Lights
☐ Beans	☐ Face Sensitivity	☐ Irritability	☐ Lack of Vision
☐ Caffeine	☐ Irritability	☐ Light-headedness	☐ Numbness FACE ARM LEG
☐ Cheese	☐ Light Sensitivity	☐ Light Sensitivity	☐ Zig Zag Lines
☐ Chocolate	☐ Neck Tightness	☐ Malaise	☐
☐ Fermented Foods	☐ Unexplained Fatigue	☐ Nasal Congestion	☐
☐ MSG	☐ Visual Disturbances	☐ Nausea/Vomiting	**TRIGGER & SYMPTOM NOTES**
☐ Non Friendly Fruits	☐	☐ Sound Sensitivity	
☐ Nuts	☐	☐ Tender Scalp	
☐ Processed Meats	☐	☐	
☐	☐	☐	
☐	☐	☐	
☐	☐		

REMEDIES

(NATURAL)		(OTC- COUNTER MEDS)	(Rx - PREVENTIVE)	(Rx - RELIEF)	(SUPPLEMENTS)
☐ Acupuncture	☐ Ice Pack	☐ Excedrin	☐ Amitriptyline	☐ Naproxin	☐ B2
☐ Acupressure	☐ Massage	☐ Ibuprofen	☐ Atenolol	☐ Nurtec	☐ Butterbur
☐ Caffeine	☐ Relaxation	☐ Tylenol	☐ Gabapentin	☐ Sumatriptan	☐ Feverfew
☐ Dark Room	☐ Silence	☐	☐ Nurtriptyline	☐ Rizatriptan	☐ Magnesium
☐ Hot Compress	☐ Walk	☐	☐ Propranolol	☐ Ubrelvy	☐
☐ Hydration	☐	☐	☐ Topamax	☐	☐
☐	☐	☐	☐ Valproate	☐	☐
☐	☐	☐	☐	WITHIN 1 HR OF PAIN YES NO	PAIN RELIEF YES NO
☐	☐	☐	☐		

REMEDY NOTES

IMPACT ON DAILY ACTIVITIES

NONE | MILD | MODERATE | SEVERE

WWW.ONEMINUTEMIGRAINEDIARY.COM

One Minute MIGRAINE Diary

Date : ______________________

Start Time : ______________ End Time : ______________ Duration : ________

PAIN SCALE [1-10]	MENSTRUAL PERIOD	PAIN TYPE	WATER
1 2 3 4 5 6 7 8 9 10 MILD MODERATE SEVERE	YES NO Birth Control Pills YES NO	Stabbing Burning Pulsating Shocking Pressure Pounding SLEEP	MISSED MEALS YES NO

PAIN LOCATION	WEATHER	STRESS
FRONT BACK LEFT RIGHT TOP	TEMP °	YES NO
	LIGHTS YES NO / SOUNDS YES NO	SMELLS YES NO

FOODS CONSUMED (within last 24 hours)	PRODROME (1-2 hours before headache)	SYMPTOMS	AURA (20-30 mins before)
☐ Alcohol	☐ Excessive Thirst	☐ Distorted Vision	☐ Black Spots
☐ Artificial Sweetener	☐ Excessive Yawning	☐ Dizziness	☐ Flashing Lights
☐ Beans	☐ Face Sensitivity	☐ Irritability	☐ Lack of Vision
☐ Caffeine	☐ Irritability	☐ Light-headedness	☐ Numbness FACE ARM LEG
☐ Cheese	☐ Light Sensitivity	☐ Light Sensitivity	☐ Zig Zag Lines
☐ Chocolate	☐ Neck Tightness	☐ Malaise	☐
☐ Fermented Foods	☐ Unexplained Fatigue	☐ Nasal Congestion	☐
☐ MSG	☐ Visual Disturbances	☐ Nausea/Vomiting	TRIGGER & SYMPTOM NOTES
☐ Non Friendly Fruits	☐	☐ Sound Sensitivity	
☐ Nuts	☐	☐ Tender Scalp	
☐ Processed Meats	☐	☐	
☐	☐	☐	
☐	☐	☐	
☐			

REMEDIES

(NATURAL)		(OTC- COUNTER MEDS)	(Rx - PREVENTIVE)	(Rx - RELIEF)	(SUPPLEMENTS)
☐ Acupuncture	☐ Ice Pack	☐ Excedrin	☐ Amitriptyline	☐ Naproxin	☐ B2
☐ Acupressure	☐ Massage	☐ Ibuprofen	☐ Atenolol	☐ Nurtec	☐ Butterbur
☐ Caffeine	☐ Relaxation	☐ Tylenol	☐ Gabapentin	☐ Sumatriptan	☐ Feverfew
☐ Dark Room	☐ Silence	☐	☐ Nurtriptyline	☐ Rizatriptan	☐ Magnesium
☐ Hot Compress	☐ Walk	☐	☐ Propranolol	☐ Ubrelvy	☐
☐ Hydration	☐	☐	☐ Topamax	☐	☐
☐	☐	☐	☐ Valproate	☐	☐
☐	☐	☐	☐	WITHIN 1 HR OF PAIN YES NO	PAIN RELIEF YES NO
☐	☐	☐	☐		

REMEDY NOTES

IMPACT ON DAILY ACTIVITIES

NONE | MILD | MODERATE | SEVERE

WWW.ONEMINUTEMIGRAINEDIARY.COM

One Minute MIGRAINE Diary

Date : ____________________

Start Time : ______________ End Time : ______________ Duration : ______

PAIN SCALE [1-10]
1 2 3 4 5 6 7 8 9 10
MILD MODERATE SEVERE

MENSTRUAL PERIOD
YES NO
Birth Control Pills
YES NO

PAIN TYPE
Stabbing Burning Pulsating Shocking Pressure Pounding

SLEEP

WATER

MISSED MEALS
YES NO

PAIN LOCATION
FRONT BACK LEFT RIGHT TOP

WEATHER
TEMP °

STRESS
YES NO

LIGHTS
YES NO

SOUNDS
YES NO

SMELLS
YES NO

FOODS CONSUMED (within last 24 hours)
- ☐ Alcohol
- ☐ Artificial Sweetener
- ☐ Beans
- ☐ Caffeine
- ☐ Cheese
- ☐ Chocolate
- ☐ Fermented Foods
- ☐ MSG
- ☐ Non Friendly Fruits
- ☐ Nuts
- ☐ Processed Meats
- ☐
- ☐
- ☐

PRODROME (1-2 hours before headache)
- ☐ Excessive Thirst
- ☐ Excessive Yawning
- ☐ Face Sensitivity
- ☐ Irritability
- ☐ Light Sensitivity
- ☐ Neck Tightness
- ☐ Unexplained Fatigue
- ☐ Visual Disturbances
- ☐
- ☐
- ☐
- ☐
- ☐

SYMPTOMS
- ☐ Distorted Vision
- ☐ Dizziness
- ☐ Irritability
- ☐ Light-headedness
- ☐ Light Sensitivity
- ☐ Malaise
- ☐ Nasal Congestion
- ☐ Nausea/Vomiting
- ☐ Sound Sensitivity
- ☐ Tender Scalp
- ☐
- ☐
- ☐

AURA (20-30 mins before)
- ☐ Black Spots
- ☐ Flashing Lights
- ☐ Lack of Vision
- ☐ Numbness FACE ARM LEG
- ☐ Zig Zag Lines
- ☐
- ☐

TRIGGER & SYMPTOM NOTES

REMEDIES

(NATURAL)
- ☐ Acupuncture
- ☐ Acupressure
- ☐ Caffeine
- ☐ Dark Room
- ☐ Hot Compress
- ☐ Hydration
- ☐
- ☐
- ☐
- ☐ Ice Pack
- ☐ Massage
- ☐ Relaxation
- ☐ Silence
- ☐ Walk
- ☐
- ☐
- ☐
- ☐

(OTC- COUNTER MEDS)
- ☐ Excedrin
- ☐ Ibuprofen
- ☐ Tylenol
- ☐
- ☐
- ☐
- ☐
- ☐
- ☐

(Rx - PREVENTIVE)
- ☐ Amitriptyline
- ☐ Atenolol
- ☐ Gabapentin
- ☐ Nurtriptyline
- ☐ Propranolol
- ☐ Topamax
- ☐ Valproate
- ☐
- ☐

(Rx - RELIEF)
- ☐ Naproxin
- ☐ Nurtec
- ☐ Sumatriptan
- ☐ Rizatriptan
- ☐ Ubrelvy
- ☐
- ☐

(SUPPLEMENTS)
- ☐ B2
- ☐ Butterbur
- ☐ Feverfew
- ☐ Magnesium
- ☐
- ☐
- ☐

WITHIN 1 HR OF PAIN YES NO PAIN RELIEF YES NO

REMEDY NOTES

IMPACT ON DAILY ACTIVITIES
NONE | MILD | MODERATE | SEVERE

WWW.ONEMINUTEMIGRAINEDIARY.COM

One Minute MIGRAINE Diary

Date : ______________________

Start Time : ______________ End Time : ____________ Duration : ______

PAIN SCALE [1-10]	MENSTRUAL PERIOD	PAIN TYPE	WATER
1 2 3 4 5 6 7 8 9 10 MILD MODERATE SEVERE	YES NO Birth Control Pills YES NO	Stabbing Burning Pulsating Shocking Pressure Pounding **SLEEP**	**MISSED MEALS** YES NO

PAIN LOCATION

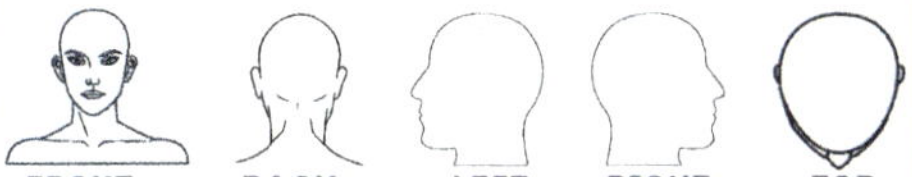

FRONT BACK LEFT RIGHT TOP

WEATHER

TEMP °

LIGHTS YES NO | **SOUNDS** YES NO

STRESS YES NO

SMELLS YES NO

FOODS CONSUMED (within last 24 hours)	PRODROME (1-2 hours before headache)	SYMPTOMS	AURA (20-30 mins before)
☐ Alcohol	☐ Excessive Thirst	☐ Distorted Vision	☐ Black Spots
☐ Artificial Sweetener	☐ Excessive Yawning	☐ Dizziness	☐ Flashing Lights
☐ Beans	☐ Face Sensitivity	☐ Irritability	☐ Lack of Vision
☐ Caffeine	☐ Irritability	☐ Light-headedness	☐ Numbness FACE ARM LEG
☐ Cheese	☐ Light Sensitivity	☐ Light Sensitivity	☐ Zig Zag Lines
☐ Chocolate	☐ Neck Tightness	☐ Malaise	☐
☐ Fermented Foods	☐ Unexplained Fatigue	☐ Nasal Congestion	☐
☐ MSG	☐ Visual Disturbances	☐ Nausea/Vomiting	**TRIGGER & SYMPTOM NOTES**
☐ Non Friendly Fruits	☐	☐ Sound Sensitivity	
☐ Nuts	☐	☐ Tender Scalp	
☐ Processed Meats	☐	☐	
☐	☐	☐	
☐	☐	☐	
☐	☐		

REMEDIES

(NATURAL)		(OTC- COUNTER MEDS)	(Rx - PREVENTIVE)	(Rx - RELIEF)	(SUPPLEMENTS)
☐ Acupuncture	☐ Ice Pack	☐ Excedrin	☐ Amitriptyline	☐ Naproxin	☐ B2
☐ Acupressure	☐ Massage	☐ Ibuprofen	☐ Atenolol	☐ Nurtec	☐ Butterbur
☐ Caffeine	☐ Relaxation	☐ Tylenol	☐ Gabapentin	☐ Sumatriptan	☐ Feverfew
☐ Dark Room	☐ Silence	☐	☐ Nurtriptyline	☐ Rizatriptan	☐ Magnesium
☐ Hot Compress	☐ Walk	☐	☐ Propranolol	☐ Ubrelvy	☐
☐ Hydration	☐	☐	☐ Topamax	☐	☐
☐	☐	☐	☐ Valproate	☐	☐
☐	☐	☐	☐	WITHIN 1 HR OF PAIN YES NO	PAIN RELIEF YES NO
☐	☐	☐	☐		

REMEDY NOTES

IMPACT ON DAILY ACTIVITIES

NONE | MILD | MODERATE | SEVERE

WWW.ONEMINUTEMIGRAINEDIARY.COM

One Minute

MIGRAINE Diary

Date : ______________________

Start Time : ______________ End Time : ______________ Duration : ________

PAIN SCALE [1-10]	MENSTRUAL PERIOD	PAIN TYPE	WATER
1 2 3 4 5 6 7 8 9 10 MILD MODERATE SEVERE	YES NO Birth Control Pills YES NO	Stabbing Burning Pulsating Shocking Pressure Pounding **SLEEP**	**MISSED MEALS** YES NO

PAIN LOCATION	WEATHER	STRESS
FRONT BACK LEFT RIGHT TOP	° TEMP	YES NO
	LIGHTS YES NO **SOUNDS** YES NO	**SMELLS** YES NO

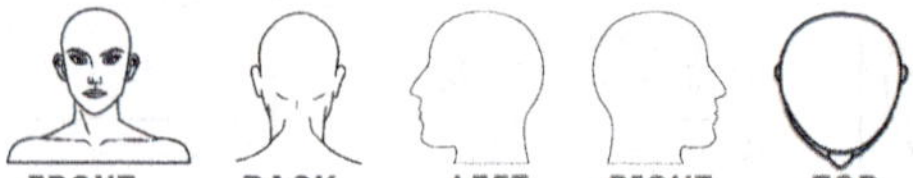

FOODS CONSUMED (within last 24 hours)	PRODROME (1-2 hours before headache)	SYMPTOMS	AURA (20-30 mins before)
☐ Alcohol	☐ Excessive Thirst	☐ Distorted Vision	☐ Black Spots
☐ Artificial Sweetener	☐ Excessive Yawning	☐ Dizziness	☐ Flashing Lights
☐ Beans	☐ Face Sensitivity	☐ Irritability	☐ Lack of Vision
☐ Caffeine	☐ Irritability	☐ Light-headedness	☐ Numbness FACE ARM LEG
☐ Cheese	☐ Light Sensitivity	☐ Light Sensitivity	☐ Zig Zag Lines
☐ Chocolate	☐ Neck Tightness	☐ Malaise	☐
☐ Fermented Foods	☐ Unexplained Fatigue	☐ Nasal Congestion	☐
☐ MSG	☐ Visual Disturbances	☐ Nausea/Vomiting	**TRIGGER & SYMPTOM NOTES**
☐ Non Friendly Fruits	☐	☐ Sound Sensitivity	
☐ Nuts	☐	☐ Tender Scalp	
☐ Processed Meats	☐	☐	
☐	☐	☐	
☐	☐	☐	
☐			

REMEDIES

(NATURAL)		(OTC- COUNTER MEDS)	(Rx - PREVENTIVE)	(Rx - RELIEF)	(SUPPLEMENTS)
☐ Acupuncture	☐ Ice Pack	☐ Excedrin	☐ Amitriptyline	☐ Naproxin	☐ B2
☐ Acupressure	☐ Massage	☐ Ibuprofen	☐ Atenolol	☐ Nurtec	☐ Butterbur
☐ Caffeine	☐ Relaxation	☐ Tylenol	☐ Gabapentin	☐ Sumatriptan	☐ Feverfew
☐ Dark Room	☐ Silence	☐	☐ Nurtriptyline	☐ Rizatriptan	☐ Magnesium
☐ Hot Compress	☐ Walk	☐	☐ Propranolol	☐ Ubrelvy	☐
☐ Hydration	☐	☐	☐ Topamax	☐	☐
☐	☐	☐	☐ Valproate	☐	☐
☐	☐	☐	☐	WITHIN 1 HR OF PAIN YES NO	PAIN RELIEF YES NO
☐	☐	☐	☐		

REMEDY NOTES

IMPACT ON DAILY ACTIVITIES

NONE | MILD | MODERATE | SEVERE

WWW.ONEMINUTEMIGRAINEDIARY.COM

One Minute MIGRAINE Diary

Date : ____________________

Start Time : ______________ End Time : ______________ Duration : ________

PAIN SCALE [1-10]	MENSTRUAL PERIOD	PAIN TYPE	WATER
1 2 3 4 5 6 7 8 9 10 MILD MODERATE SEVERE	YES NO Birth Control Pills YES NO	Stabbing Burning Pulsating Shocking Pressure Pounding SLEEP	MISSED MEALS YES NO
PAIN LOCATION FRONT BACK LEFT RIGHT TOP		WEATHER TEMP °	STRESS YES NO
		LIGHTS YES NO SOUNDS YES NO	SMELLS YES NO

FOODS CONSUMED (within last 24 hours)	PRODROME (1-2 hours before headache)	SYMPTOMS	AURA (20-30 mins before)
☐ Alcohol	☐ Excessive Thirst	☐ Distorted Vision	☐ Black Spots
☐ Artificial Sweetener	☐ Excessive Yawning	☐ Dizziness	☐ Flashing Lights
☐ Beans	☐ Face Sensitivity	☐ Irritability	☐ Lack of Vision
☐ Caffeine	☐ Irritability	☐ Light-headedness	☐ Numbness FACE ARM LEG
☐ Cheese	☐ Light Sensitivity	☐ Light Sensitivity	☐ Zig Zag Lines
☐ Chocolate	☐ Neck Tightness	☐ Malaise	☐
☐ Fermented Foods	☐ Unexplained Fatigue	☐ Nasal Congestion	☐
☐ MSG	☐ Visual Disturbances	☐ Nausea/Vomiting	TRIGGER & SYMPTOM NOTES
☐ Non Friendly Fruits	☐	☐ Sound Sensitivity	
☐ Nuts	☐	☐ Tender Scalp	
☐ Processed Meats	☐	☐	
☐	☐	☐	
☐	☐	☐	
☐	☐		

REMEDIES

(NATURAL)		(OTC- COUNTER MEDS)	(Rx - PREVENTIVE)	(Rx - RELIEF)	(SUPPLEMENTS)
☐ Acupuncture	☐ Ice Pack	☐ Excedrin	☐ Amitriptyline	☐ Naproxin	☐ B2
☐ Acupressure	☐ Massage	☐ Ibuprofen	☐ Atenolol	☐ Nurtec	☐ Butterbur
☐ Caffeine	☐ Relaxation	☐ Tylenol	☐ Gabapentin	☐ Sumatriptan	☐ Feverfew
☐ Dark Room	☐ Silence	☐	☐ Nurtriptyline	☐ Rizatriptan	☐ Magnesium
☐ Hot Compress	☐ Walk	☐	☐ Propranolol	☐ Ubrelvy	☐
☐ Hydration	☐	☐	☐ Topamax	☐	☐
☐	☐	☐	☐ Valproate	☐	☐
☐	☐	☐	☐	WITHIN 1 HR OF PAIN YES NO	PAIN RELIEF YES NO
☐	☐	☐	☐		

REMEDY NOTES

IMPACT ON DAILY ACTIVITIES

NONE | MILD | MODERATE | SEVERE

WWW.ONEMINUTEMIGRAINEDIARY.COM

One Minute MIGRAINE Diary

Date : ____________________

Start Time : ______________ End Time : ____________ Duration : ________

PAIN SCALE [1-10]	MENSTRUAL PERIOD	PAIN TYPE	WATER
1 2 3 4 5 6 7 8 9 10 MILD MODERATE SEVERE	YES NO Birth Control Pills YES NO	Stabbing Burning Pulsating Shocking Pressure Pounding SLEEP	MISSED MEALS YES NO

PAIN LOCATION	WEATHER	STRESS
FRONT BACK LEFT RIGHT TOP	° TEMP	YES NO
	LIGHTS YES NO / SOUNDS YES NO	SMELLS YES NO

FOODS CONSUMED (within last 24 hours)	PRODROME (1-2 hours before headache)	SYMPTOMS	AURA (20-30 mins before)
☐ Alcohol	☐ Excessive Thirst	☐ Distorted Vision	☐ Black Spots
☐ Artificial Sweetener	☐ Excessive Yawning	☐ Dizziness	☐ Flashing Lights
☐ Beans	☐ Face Sensitivity	☐ Irritability	☐ Lack of Vision
☐ Caffeine	☐ Irritability	☐ Light-headedness	☐ Numbness FACE ARM LEG
☐ Cheese	☐ Light Sensitivity	☐ Light Sensitivity	☐ Zig Zag Lines
☐ Chocolate	☐ Neck Tightness	☐ Malaise	☐
☐ Fermented Foods	☐ Unexplained Fatigue	☐ Nasal Congestion	☐
☐ MSG	☐ Visual Disturbances	☐ Nausea/Vomiting	TRIGGER & SYMPTOM NOTES
☐ Non Friendly Fruits	☐	☐ Sound Sensitivity	
☐ Nuts	☐	☐ Tender Scalp	
☐ Processed Meats	☐	☐	
☐	☐	☐	
☐	☐	☐	
☐			

REMEDIES

(NATURAL)		(OTC- COUNTER MEDS)	(Rx - PREVENTIVE)	(Rx - RELIEF)	(SUPPLEMENTS)
☐ Acupuncture	☐ Ice Pack	☐ Excedrin	☐ Amitriptyline	☐ Naproxin	☐ B2
☐ Acupressure	☐ Massage	☐ Ibuprofen	☐ Atenolol	☐ Nurtec	☐ Butterbur
☐ Caffeine	☐ Relaxation	☐ Tylenol	☐ Gabapentin	☐ Sumatriptan	☐ Feverfew
☐ Dark Room	☐ Silence	☐	☐ Nurtriptyline	☐ Rizatriptan	☐ Magnesium
☐ Hot Compress	☐ Walk	☐	☐ Propranolol	☐ Ubrelvy	☐
☐ Hydration	☐	☐	☐ Topamax	☐	☐
☐	☐	☐	☐ Valproate	☐	☐
☐	☐	☐	☐	WITHIN 1 HR OF PAIN YES NO	PAIN RELIEF YES NO
☐	☐	☐	☐		

REMEDY NOTES

IMPACT ON DAILY ACTIVITIES

NONE | MILD | MODERATE | SEVERE

WWW.ONEMINUTEMIGRAINEDIARY.COM

One Minute MIGRAINE Diary

Date : ____________________

Start Time : ______________ End Time : ____________ Duration : ________

PAIN SCALE [1-10]	MENSTRUAL PERIOD	PAIN TYPE	WATER
1 2 3 4 5 6 7 8 9 10 MILD MODERATE SEVERE	YES NO Birth Control Pills YES NO	Stabbing Burning Pulsating Shocking Pressure Pounding SLEEP	MISSED MEALS YES NO
PAIN LOCATION FRONT BACK LEFT RIGHT TOP		WEATHER TEMP °	STRESS YES NO
		LIGHTS YES NO SOUNDS YES NO	SMELLS YES NO

FOODS CONSUMED (within last 24 hours)	PRODROME (1-2 hours before headache)	SYMPTOMS	AURA (20-30 mins before)
☐ Alcohol	☐ Excessive Thirst	☐ Distorted Vision	☐ Black Spots
☐ Artificial Sweetener	☐ Excessive Yawning	☐ Dizziness	☐ Flashing Lights
☐ Beans	☐ Face Sensitivity	☐ Irritability	☐ Lack of Vision
☐ Caffeine	☐ Irritability	☐ Light-headedness	☐ Numbness FACE ARM LEG
☐ Cheese	☐ Light Sensitivity	☐ Light Sensitivity	☐ Zig Zag Lines
☐ Chocolate	☐ Neck Tightness	☐ Malaise	☐
☐ Fermented Foods	☐ Unexplained Fatigue	☐ Nasal Congestion	☐
☐ MSG	☐ Visual Disturbances	☐ Nausea/Vomiting	TRIGGER & SYMPTOM NOTES
☐ Non Friendly Fruits	☐	☐ Sound Sensitivity	
☐ Nuts	☐	☐ Tender Scalp	
☐ Processed Meats	☐	☐	
☐	☐	☐	
☐	☐	☐	
☐			

REMEDIES

(NATURAL)		(OTC- COUNTER MEDS)	(Rx - PREVENTIVE)	(Rx - RELIEF)	(SUPPLEMENTS)
☐ Acupuncture	☐ Ice Pack	☐ Excedrin	☐ Amitriptyline	☐ Naproxin	☐ B2
☐ Acupressure	☐ Massage	☐ Ibuprofen	☐ Atenolol	☐ Nurtec	☐ Butterbur
☐ Caffeine	☐ Relaxation	☐ Tylenol	☐ Gabapentin	☐ Sumatriptan	☐ Feverfew
☐ Dark Room	☐ Silence	☐	☐ Nurtriptyline	☐ Rizatriptan	☐ Magnesium
☐ Hot Compress	☐ Walk	☐	☐ Propranolol	☐ Ubrelvy	☐
☐ Hydration	☐	☐	☐ Topamax	☐	☐
☐	☐	☐	☐ Valproate	☐	☐
☐	☐	☐	☐	WITHIN 1 HR OF PAIN YES NO	PAIN RELIEF YES NO
☐	☐	☐	☐		

REMEDY NOTES

IMPACT ON DAILY ACTIVITIES

NONE | MILD | MODERATE | SEVERE

WWW.ONEMINUTEMIGRAINEDIARY.COM

One Minute MIGRAINE Diary

Date : ____________________

Start Time : ______________ End Time : ____________ Duration : ______

PAIN SCALE [1-10]	MENSTRUAL PERIOD	PAIN TYPE	WATER
1 2 3 4 5 6 7 8 9 10 MILD MODERATE SEVERE	YES NO Birth Control Pills YES NO	Stabbing Burning Pulsating Shocking Pressure Pounding **SLEEP**	**MISSED MEALS** YES NO
PAIN LOCATION FRONT BACK LEFT RIGHT TOP		**WEATHER** ° TEMP	**STRESS** YES NO
		LIGHTS YES NO **SOUNDS** YES NO	**SMELLS** YES NO

FOODS CONSUMED (within last 24 hours)	PRODROME (1-2 hours before headache)	SYMPTOMS	AURA (20-30 mins before)
☐ Alcohol	☐ Excessive Thirst	☐ Distorted Vision	☐ Black Spots
☐ Artificial Sweetener	☐ Excessive Yawning	☐ Dizziness	☐ Flashing Lights
☐ Beans	☐ Face Sensitivity	☐ Irritability	☐ Lack of Vision
☐ Caffeine	☐ Irritability	☐ Light-headedness	☐ Numbness FACE ARM LEG
☐ Cheese	☐ Light Sensitivity	☐ Light Sensitivity	☐ Zig Zag Lines
☐ Chocolate	☐ Neck Tightness	☐ Malaise	☐
☐ Fermented Foods	☐ Unexplained Fatigue	☐ Nasal Congestion	☐
☐ MSG	☐ Visual Disturbances	☐ Nausea/Vomiting	TRIGGER & SYMPTOM NOTES
☐ Non Friendly Fruits	☐	☐ Sound Sensitivity	
☐ Nuts	☐	☐ Tender Scalp	
☐ Processed Meats	☐	☐	
☐	☐	☐	
☐	☐	☐	
☐			

REMEDIES

(NATURAL)		(OTC- COUNTER MEDS)	(Rx - PREVENTIVE)	(Rx - RELIEF)	(SUPPLEMENTS)
☐ Acupuncture	☐ Ice Pack	☐ Excedrin	☐ Amitriptyline	☐ Naproxin	☐ B2
☐ Acupressure	☐ Massage	☐ Ibuprofen	☐ Atenolol	☐ Nurtec	☐ Butterbur
☐ Caffeine	☐ Relaxation	☐ Tylenol	☐ Gabapentin	☐ Sumatriptan	☐ Feverfew
☐ Dark Room	☐ Silence	☐	☐ Nurtriptyline	☐ Rizatriptan	☐ Magnesium
☐ Hot Compress	☐ Walk	☐	☐ Propranolol	☐ Ubrelvy	☐
☐ Hydration	☐	☐	☐ Topamax	☐	☐
☐	☐	☐	☐ Valproate	☐	☐
☐	☐	☐	☐	WITHIN 1 HR OF PAIN YES NO	PAIN RELIEF YES NO
☐	☐	☐	☐		

REMEDY NOTES

IMPACT ON DAILY ACTIVITIES

NONE | MILD | MODERATE | SEVERE

One Minute MIGRAINE Diary

Date : ____________________

Start Time : ______________ End Time : ____________ Duration : ______

PAIN SCALE [1-10]

1 2 3 4 5 6 7 8 9 10

MILD MODERATE SEVERE

MENSTRUAL PERIOD

YES NO

Birth Control Pills

YES NO

PAIN TYPE

Stabbing Burning Pulsating Shocking Pressure Pounding

SLEEP

WATER

MISSED MEALS

YES NO

PAIN LOCATION

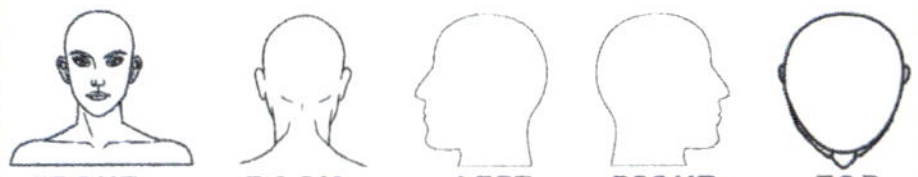

FRONT BACK LEFT RIGHT TOP

WEATHER

TEMP °

STRESS

YES NO

LIGHTS

YES NO

SOUNDS

YES NO

SMELLS

YES NO

FOODS CONSUMED (within last 24 hours)	PRODROME (1-2 hours before headache)	SYMPTOMS	AURA (20-30 mins before)
☐ Alcohol	☐ Excessive Thirst	☐ Distorted Vision	☐ Black Spots
☐ Artificial Sweetener	☐ Excessive Yawning	☐ Dizziness	☐ Flashing Lights
☐ Beans	☐ Face Sensitivity	☐ Irritability	☐ Lack of Vision
☐ Caffeine	☐ Irritability	☐ Light-headedness	☐ Numbness FACE ARM LEG
☐ Cheese	☐ Light Sensitivity	☐ Light Sensitivity	☐ Zig Zag Lines
☐ Chocolate	☐ Neck Tightness	☐ Malaise	☐
☐ Fermented Foods	☐ Unexplained Fatigue	☐ Nasal Congestion	☐
☐ MSG	☐ Visual Disturbances	☐ Nausea/Vomiting	**TRIGGER & SYMPTOM NOTES**
☐ Non Friendly Fruits	☐	☐ Sound Sensitivity	
☐ Nuts	☐	☐ Tender Scalp	
☐ Processed Meats	☐	☐	
☐	☐	☐	
☐	☐	☐	
☐	☐		

REMEDIES

(NATURAL)		(OTC- COUNTER MEDS)	(Rx - PREVENTIVE)	(Rx - RELIEF)	(SUPPLEMENTS)
☐ Acupuncture	☐ Ice Pack	☐ Excedrin	☐ Amitriptyline	☐ Naproxin	☐ B2
☐ Acupressure	☐ Massage	☐ Ibuprofen	☐ Atenolol	☐ Nurtec	☐ Butterbur
☐ Caffeine	☐ Relaxation	☐ Tylenol	☐ Gabapentin	☐ Sumatriptan	☐ Feverfew
☐ Dark Room	☐ Silence	☐	☐ Nurtriptyline	☐ Rizatriptan	☐ Magnesium
☐ Hot Compress	☐ Walk	☐	☐ Propranolol	☐ Ubrelvy	☐
☐ Hydration	☐	☐	☐ Topamax	☐	☐
☐	☐	☐	☐ Valproate	☐	☐
☐	☐	☐	☐	WITHIN 1 HR OF PAIN YES NO	PAIN RELIEF YES NO
☐	☐	☐	☐		

REMEDY NOTES

IMPACT ON DAILY ACTIVITIES

NONE | MILD | MODERATE | SEVERE

WWW.ONEMINUTEMIGRAINEDIARY.COM

One Minute MIGRAINE Diary

Date : ____________________

Start Time : ______________ End Time : ______________ Duration : ________

PAIN SCALE [1-10]	MENSTRUAL PERIOD	PAIN TYPE	WATER
1 2 3 4 5 6 7 8 9 10 MILD MODERATE SEVERE	YES NO Birth Control Pills YES NO	Stabbing Burning Pulsating Shocking Pressure Pounding SLEEP	MISSED MEALS YES NO
PAIN LOCATION FRONT BACK LEFT RIGHT TOP		WEATHER TEMP	STRESS YES NO
		LIGHTS YES NO SOUNDS YES NO	SMELLS YES NO

FOODS CONSUMED (within last 24 hours)	PRODROME (1-2 hours before headache)	SYMPTOMS	AURA (20-30 mins before)
☐ Alcohol	☐ Excessive Thirst	☐ Distorted Vision	☐ Black Spots
☐ Artificial Sweetener	☐ Excessive Yawning	☐ Dizziness	☐ Flashing Lights
☐ Beans	☐ Face Sensitivity	☐ Irritability	☐ Lack of Vision
☐ Caffeine	☐ Irritability	☐ Light-headedness	☐ Numbness FACE ARM LEG
☐ Cheese	☐ Light Sensitivity	☐ Light Sensitivity	☐ Zig Zag Lines
☐ Chocolate	☐ Neck Tightness	☐ Malaise	☐
☐ Fermented Foods	☐ Unexplained Fatigue	☐ Nasal Congestion	☐
☐ MSG	☐ Visual Disturbances	☐ Nausea/Vomiting	TRIGGER & SYMPTOM NOTES
☐ Non Friendly Fruits	☐	☐ Sound Sensitivity	
☐ Nuts	☐	☐ Tender Scalp	
☐ Processed Meats	☐	☐	
☐	☐	☐	
☐	☐	☐	
☐			

REMEDIES

(NATURAL)		(OTC- COUNTER MEDS)	(Rx - PREVENTIVE)	(Rx - RELIEF)	(SUPPLEMENTS)
☐ Acupuncture	☐ Ice Pack	☐ Excedrin	☐ Amitriptyline	☐ Naproxin	☐ B2
☐ Acupressure	☐ Massage	☐ Ibuprofen	☐ Atenolol	☐ Nurtec	☐ Butterbur
☐ Caffeine	☐ Relaxation	☐ Tylenol	☐ Gabapentin	☐ Sumatriptan	☐ Feverfew
☐ Dark Room	☐ Silence	☐	☐ Nurtriptyline	☐ Rizatriptan	☐ Magnesium
☐ Hot Compress	☐ Walk	☐	☐ Propranolol	☐ Ubrelvy	☐
☐ Hydration	☐	☐	☐ Topamax	☐	☐
☐	☐	☐	☐ Valproate	☐	☐
☐	☐	☐	☐	WITHIN 1 HR OF PAIN YES NO	PAIN RELIEF YES NO
☐	☐	☐	☐		

REMEDY NOTES

IMPACT ON DAILY ACTIVITIES

NONE | MILD | MODERATE | SEVERE

WWW.ONEMINUTEMIGRAINEDIARY.COM

One Minute MIGRAINE Diary

Date : ______________________

Start Time : ______________ End Time : ______________ Duration : ________

PAIN SCALE [1-10]	MENSTRUAL PERIOD	PAIN TYPE	WATER
1 2 3 4 5 6 7 8 9 10 MILD MODERATE SEVERE	YES NO Birth Control Pills YES NO	Stabbing Burning Pulsating Shocking Pressure Pounding **SLEEP**	**MISSED MEALS** YES NO

PAIN LOCATION	WEATHER	STRESS
FRONT BACK LEFT RIGHT TOP	TEMP °	YES NO
	LIGHTS YES NO **SOUNDS** YES NO	**SMELLS** YES NO

FOODS CONSUMED (within last 24 hours)	PRODROME (1-2 hours before headache)	SYMPTOMS	AURA (20-30 mins before)
☐ Alcohol	☐ Excessive Thirst	☐ Distorted Vision	☐ Black Spots
☐ Artificial Sweetener	☐ Excessive Yawning	☐ Dizziness	☐ Flashing Lights
☐ Beans	☐ Face Sensitivity	☐ Irritability	☐ Lack of Vision
☐ Caffeine	☐ Irritability	☐ Light-headedness	☐ Numbness FACE ARM LEG
☐ Cheese	☐ Light Sensitivity	☐ Light Sensitivity	☐ Zig Zag Lines
☐ Chocolate	☐ Neck Tightness	☐ Malaise	☐
☐ Fermented Foods	☐ Unexplained Fatigue	☐ Nasal Congestion	☐
☐ MSG	☐ Visual Disturbances	☐ Nausea/Vomiting	**TRIGGER & SYMPTOM NOTES**
☐ Non Friendly Fruits	☐	☐ Sound Sensitivity	
☐ Nuts	☐	☐ Tender Scalp	
☐ Processed Meats	☐	☐	
☐	☐	☐	
☐	☐	☐	
☐	☐		

REMEDIES

(NATURAL)		(OTC- COUNTER MEDS)	(Rx - PREVENTIVE)	(Rx - RELIEF)	(SUPPLEMENTS)
☐ Acupuncture	☐ Ice Pack	☐ Excedrin	☐ Amitriptyline	☐ Naproxin	☐ B2
☐ Acupressure	☐ Massage	☐ Ibuprofen	☐ Atenolol	☐ Nurtec	☐ Butterbur
☐ Caffeine	☐ Relaxation	☐ Tylenol	☐ Gabapentin	☐ Sumatriptan	☐ Feverfew
☐ Dark Room	☐ Silence	☐	☐ Nurtriptyline	☐ Rizatriptan	☐ Magnesium
☐ Hot Compress	☐ Walk	☐	☐ Propranolol	☐ Ubrelvy	☐
☐ Hydration	☐	☐	☐ Topamax	☐	☐
☐	☐	☐	☐ Valproate	☐	☐
☐	☐	☐	☐	WITHIN 1 HR OF PAIN YES NO	PAIN RELIEF YES NO
☐	☐	☐	☐		

REMEDY NOTES

IMPACT ON DAILY ACTIVITIES

NONE | MILD | MODERATE | SEVERE

WWW.ONEMINUTEMIGRAINEDIARY.COM

One Minute MIGRAINE Diary

Date : ____________________

Start Time : ______________ End Time : ____________ Duration : ________

PAIN SCALE [1-10]

|-----|-----|-----|-----|-----|-----|-----|-----|-----|
1 2 3 4 5 6 7 8 9 10
MILD MODERATE SEVERE

MENSTRUAL PERIOD

YES NO

Birth Control Pills

YES NO

PAIN TYPE

Stabbing Burning Pulsating Shocking Pressure Pounding

SLEEP

WATER

MISSED MEALS

YES NO

PAIN LOCATION

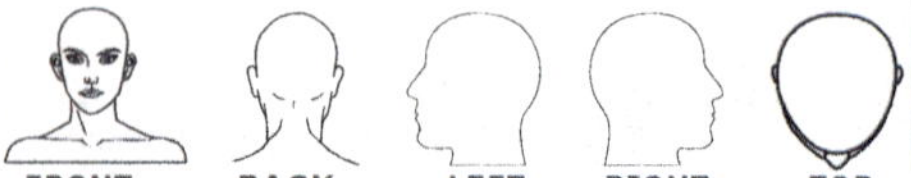

FRONT BACK LEFT RIGHT TOP

WEATHER

TEMP °

STRESS

YES NO

LIGHTS

YES NO

SOUNDS

YES NO

SMELLS

YES NO

FOODS CONSUMED (within last 24 hours)

- ☐ Alcohol
- ☐ Artificial Sweetener
- ☐ Beans
- ☐ Caffeine
- ☐ Cheese
- ☐ Chocolate
- ☐ Fermented Foods
- ☐ MSG
- ☐ Non Friendly Fruits
- ☐ Nuts
- ☐ Processed Meats
- ☐
- ☐
- ☐

PRODROME (1-2 hours before headache)

- ☐ Excessive Thirst
- ☐ Excessive Yawning
- ☐ Face Sensitivity
- ☐ Irritability
- ☐ Light Sensitivity
- ☐ Neck Tightness
- ☐ Unexplained Fatigue
- ☐ Visual Disturbances
- ☐
- ☐
- ☐
- ☐
- ☐

SYMPTOMS

- ☐ Distorted Vision
- ☐ Dizziness
- ☐ Irritability
- ☐ Light-headedness
- ☐ Light Sensitivity
- ☐ Malaise
- ☐ Nasal Congestion
- ☐ Nausea/Vomiting
- ☐ Sound Sensitivity
- ☐ Tender Scalp
- ☐
- ☐
- ☐

AURA (20-30 mins before)

- ☐ Black Spots
- ☐ Flashing Lights
- ☐ Lack of Vision
- ☐ Numbness FACE ARM LEG
- ☐ Zig Zag Lines
- ☐
- ☐

TRIGGER & SYMPTOM NOTES

REMEDIES

(NATURAL)

- ☐ Acupuncture
- ☐ Acupressure
- ☐ Caffeine
- ☐ Dark Room
- ☐ Hot Compress
- ☐ Hydration
- ☐
- ☐
- ☐
- ☐ Ice Pack
- ☐ Massage
- ☐ Relaxation
- ☐ Silence
- ☐ Walk
- ☐
- ☐
- ☐
- ☐

(OTC- COUNTER MEDS)

- ☐ Excedrin
- ☐ Ibuprofen
- ☐ Tylenol
- ☐
- ☐
- ☐
- ☐
- ☐
- ☐

(Rx - PREVENTIVE)

- ☐ Amitriptyline
- ☐ Atenolol
- ☐ Gabapentin
- ☐ Nurtriptyline
- ☐ Propranolol
- ☐ Topamax
- ☐ Valproate
- ☐
- ☐

(Rx - RELIEF)

- ☐ Naproxin
- ☐ Nurtec
- ☐ Sumatriptan
- ☐ Rizatriptan
- ☐ Ubrelvy
- ☐
- ☐

(SUPPLEMENTS)

- ☐ B2
- ☐ Butterbur
- ☐ Feverfew
- ☐ Magnesium
- ☐
- ☐
- ☐

WITHIN 1 HR OF PAIN YES NO PAIN RELIEF YES NO

REMEDY NOTES

IMPACT ON DAILY ACTIVITIES

NONE | MILD | MODERATE | SEVERE

WWW.ONEMINUTEMIGRAINEDIARY.COM

One Minute MIGRAINE Diary

Date : ____________________

Start Time : ______________ End Time : ______________ Duration : ________

PAIN SCALE [1-10]

|-----|-----|-----|-----|-----|-----|-----|-----|-----|
1 2 3 4 5 6 7 8 9 10
MILD MODERATE SEVERE

MENSTRUAL PERIOD
YES NO
Birth Control Pills
YES NO

PAIN TYPE
Stabbing Burning Pulsating Shocking Pressure Pounding

SLEEP

WATER

MISSED MEALS
YES NO

PAIN LOCATION

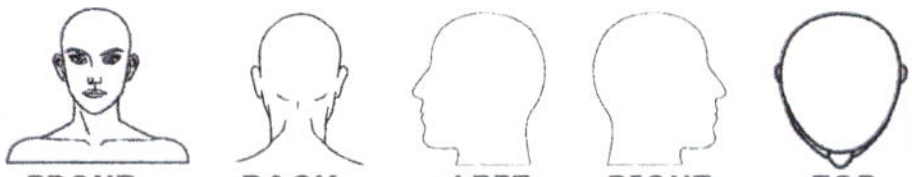

FRONT BACK LEFT RIGHT TOP

WEATHER

° TEMP

STRESS
YES NO

LIGHTS
YES NO

SOUNDS
YES NO

SMELLS
YES NO

FOODS CONSUMED (within last 24 hours)

- ☐ Alcohol
- ☐ Artificial Sweetener
- ☐ Beans
- ☐ Caffeine
- ☐ Cheese
- ☐ Chocolate
- ☐ Fermented Foods
- ☐ MSG
- ☐ Non Friendly Fruits
- ☐ Nuts
- ☐ Processed Meats
- ☐
- ☐
- ☐

PRODROME (1-2 hours before headache)

- ☐ Excessive Thirst
- ☐ Excessive Yawning
- ☐ Face Sensitivity
- ☐ Irritability
- ☐ Light Sensitivity
- ☐ Neck Tightness
- ☐ Unexplained Fatigue
- ☐ Visual Disturbances
- ☐
- ☐
- ☐
- ☐
- ☐

SYMPTOMS

- ☐ Distorted Vision
- ☐ Dizziness
- ☐ Irritability
- ☐ Light-headedness
- ☐ Light Sensitivity
- ☐ Malaise
- ☐ Nasal Congestion
- ☐ Nausea/Vomiting
- ☐ Sound Sensitivity
- ☐ Tender Scalp
- ☐
- ☐
- ☐

AURA (20-30 mins before)

- ☐ Black Spots
- ☐ Flashing Lights
- ☐ Lack of Vision
- ☐ Numbness FACE ARM LEG
- ☐ Zig Zag Lines
- ☐
- ☐

TRIGGER & SYMPTOM NOTES

REMEDIES

(NATURAL)

- ☐ Acupuncture
- ☐ Acupressure
- ☐ Caffeine
- ☐ Dark Room
- ☐ Hot Compress
- ☐ Hydration
- ☐
- ☐
- ☐
- ☐ Ice Pack
- ☐ Massage
- ☐ Relaxation
- ☐ Silence
- ☐ Walk
- ☐
- ☐
- ☐
- ☐

(OTC- COUNTER MEDS)

- ☐ Excedrin
- ☐ Ibuprofen
- ☐ Tylenol
- ☐
- ☐
- ☐
- ☐
- ☐
- ☐

(Rx - PREVENTIVE)

- ☐ Amitriptyline
- ☐ Atenolol
- ☐ Gabapentin
- ☐ Nurtriptyline
- ☐ Propranolol
- ☐ Topamax
- ☐ Valproate
- ☐
- ☐

(Rx - RELIEF)

- ☐ Naproxin
- ☐ Nurtec
- ☐ Sumatriptan
- ☐ Rizatriptan
- ☐ Ubrelvy
- ☐
- ☐

(SUPPLEMENTS)

- ☐ B2
- ☐ Butterbur
- ☐ Feverfew
- ☐ Magnesium
- ☐
- ☐
- ☐

WITHIN 1 HR OF PAIN YES NO

PAIN RELIEF YES NO

REMEDY NOTES

IMPACT ON DAILY ACTIVITIES
NONE | MILD | MODERATE | SEVERE

WWW.ONEMINUTEMIGRAINEDIARY.COM

One Minute
MIGRAINE Diary

Date : ____________________

Start Time : ______________ End Time : ______________ Duration : ________

PAIN SCALE [1-10]

1 2 3 4 5 6 7 8 9 10

MILD MODERATE SEVERE

MENSTRUAL PERIOD

YES NO

Birth Control Pills

YES NO

PAIN TYPE

Stabbing Burning Pulsating Shocking Pressure Pounding

SLEEP

WATER

MISSED MEALS

YES NO

PAIN LOCATION

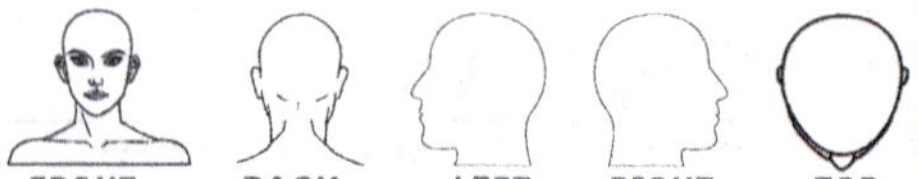

FRONT BACK LEFT RIGHT TOP

WEATHER

TEMP °

STRESS

YES NO

LIGHTS

YES NO

SOUNDS

YES NO

SMELLS

YES NO

FOODS CONSUMED (within last 24 hours)

- ☐ Alcohol
- ☐ Artificial Sweetener
- ☐ Beans
- ☐ Caffeine
- ☐ Cheese
- ☐ Chocolate
- ☐ Fermented Foods
- ☐ MSG
- ☐ Non Friendly Fruits
- ☐ Nuts
- ☐ Processed Meats
- ☐
- ☐
- ☐

PRODROME (1-2 hours before headache)

- ☐ Excessive Thirst
- ☐ Excessive Yawning
- ☐ Face Sensitivity
- ☐ Irritability
- ☐ Light Sensitivity
- ☐ Neck Tightness
- ☐ Unexplained Fatigue
- ☐ Visual Disturbances
- ☐
- ☐
- ☐
- ☐
- ☐

SYMPTOMS

- ☐ Distorted Vision
- ☐ Dizziness
- ☐ Irritability
- ☐ Light-headedness
- ☐ Light Sensitivity
- ☐ Malaise
- ☐ Nasal Congestion
- ☐ Nausea/Vomiting
- ☐ Sound Sensitivity
- ☐ Tender Scalp
- ☐
- ☐
- ☐

AURA (20-30 mins before)

- ☐ Black Spots
- ☐ Flashing Lights
- ☐ Lack of Vision
- ☐ Numbness FACE ARM LEG
- ☐ Zig Zag Lines
- ☐
- ☐

TRIGGER & SYMPTOM NOTES

REMEDIES

(NATURAL)

- ☐ Acupuncture
- ☐ Acupressure
- ☐ Caffeine
- ☐ Dark Room
- ☐ Hot Compress
- ☐ Hydration
- ☐
- ☐
- ☐
- ☐ Ice Pack
- ☐ Massage
- ☐ Relaxation
- ☐ Silence
- ☐ Walk
- ☐
- ☐
- ☐
- ☐

(OTC- COUNTER MEDS)

- ☐ Excedrin
- ☐ Ibuprofen
- ☐ Tylenol
- ☐
- ☐
- ☐
- ☐
- ☐
- ☐

(Rx - PREVENTIVE)

- ☐ Amitriptyline
- ☐ Atenolol
- ☐ Gabapentin
- ☐ Nurtriptyline
- ☐ Propranolol
- ☐ Topamax
- ☐ Valproate
- ☐
- ☐

(Rx - RELIEF)

- ☐ Naproxin
- ☐ Nurtec
- ☐ Sumatriptan
- ☐ Rizatriptan
- ☐ Ubrelvy
- ☐
- ☐

(SUPPLEMENTS)

- ☐ B2
- ☐ Butterbur
- ☐ Feverfew
- ☐ Magnesium
- ☐
- ☐
- ☐

WITHIN 1 HR OF PAIN YES NO

PAIN RELIEF YES NO

REMEDY NOTES

IMPACT ON DAILY ACTIVITIES

NONE | MILD | MODERATE | SEVERE

WWW.ONEMINUTEMIGRAINEDIARY.COM

One Minute MIGRAINE Diary

Date : ____________________

Start Time : ____________ End Time : ____________ Duration : ________

PAIN SCALE [1-10]	MENSTRUAL PERIOD	PAIN TYPE	WATER
1 2 3 4 5 6 7 8 9 10 MILD MODERATE SEVERE	YES NO Birth Control Pills YES NO	Stabbing Burning Pulsating Shocking Pressure Pounding SLEEP	MISSED MEALS YES NO

PAIN LOCATION	WEATHER	STRESS
FRONT BACK LEFT RIGHT TOP	TEMP °	YES NO
	LIGHTS YES NO / SOUNDS YES NO	SMELLS YES NO

FOODS CONSUMED (within last 24 hours)	PRODROME (1-2 hours before headache)	SYMPTOMS	AURA (20-30 mins before)
☐ Alcohol	☐ Excessive Thirst	☐ Distorted Vision	☐ Black Spots
☐ Artificial Sweetener	☐ Excessive Yawning	☐ Dizziness	☐ Flashing Lights
☐ Beans	☐ Face Sensitivity	☐ Irritability	☐ Lack of Vision
☐ Caffeine	☐ Irritability	☐ Light-headedness	☐ Numbness FACE ARM LEG
☐ Cheese	☐ Light Sensitivity	☐ Light Sensitivity	☐ Zig Zag Lines
☐ Chocolate	☐ Neck Tightness	☐ Malaise	☐
☐ Fermented Foods	☐ Unexplained Fatigue	☐ Nasal Congestion	☐
☐ MSG	☐ Visual Disturbances	☐ Nausea/Vomiting	TRIGGER & SYMPTOM NOTES
☐ Non Friendly Fruits	☐	☐ Sound Sensitivity	
☐ Nuts	☐	☐ Tender Scalp	
☐ Processed Meats	☐	☐	
☐	☐	☐	
☐	☐	☐	
☐			

REMEDIES

(NATURAL)		(OTC- COUNTER MEDS)	(Rx - PREVENTIVE)	(Rx - RELIEF)	(SUPPLEMENTS)
☐ Acupuncture	☐ Ice Pack	☐ Excedrin	☐ Amitriptyline	☐ Naproxin	☐ B2
☐ Acupressure	☐ Massage	☐ Ibuprofen	☐ Atenolol	☐ Nurtec	☐ Butterbur
☐ Caffeine	☐ Relaxation	☐ Tylenol	☐ Gabapentin	☐ Sumatriptan	☐ Feverfew
☐ Dark Room	☐ Silence	☐	☐ Nurtriptyline	☐ Rizatriptan	☐ Magnesium
☐ Hot Compress	☐ Walk	☐	☐ Propranolol	☐ Ubrelvy	☐
☐ Hydration	☐	☐	☐ Topamax	☐	☐
☐	☐	☐	☐ Valproate	☐	☐
☐	☐	☐	☐	WITHIN 1 HR OF PAIN YES NO	PAIN RELIEF YES NO
☐	☐	☐	☐		

REMEDY NOTES

IMPACT ON DAILY ACTIVITIES

NONE | MILD | MODERATE | SEVERE

WWW.ONEMINUTEMIGRAINEDIARY.COM

One Minute MIGRAINE Diary

Date : ____________________

Start Time : ____________ End Time : ____________ Duration : ________

PAIN SCALE [1-10]

1 2 3 4 5 6 7 8 9 10

MILD MODERATE SEVERE

MENSTRUAL PERIOD

YES NO

Birth Control Pills

YES NO

PAIN TYPE

Stabbing Burning Pulsating Shocking Pressure Pounding

SLEEP

WATER

MISSED MEALS

YES NO

PAIN LOCATION

FRONT BACK LEFT RIGHT TOP

WEATHER

TEMP °

STRESS

YES NO

LIGHTS

YES NO

SOUNDS

YES NO

SMELLS

YES NO

FOODS CONSUMED (within last 24 hours)

- ☐ Alcohol
- ☐ Artificial Sweetener
- ☐ Beans
- ☐ Caffeine
- ☐ Cheese
- ☐ Chocolate
- ☐ Fermented Foods
- ☐ MSG
- ☐ Non Friendly Fruits
- ☐ Nuts
- ☐ Processed Meats
- ☐
- ☐
- ☐

PRODROME (1-2 hours before headache)

- ☐ Excessive Thirst
- ☐ Excessive Yawning
- ☐ Face Sensitivity
- ☐ Irritability
- ☐ Light Sensitivity
- ☐ Neck Tightness
- ☐ Unexplained Fatigue
- ☐ Visual Disturbances
- ☐
- ☐
- ☐
- ☐
- ☐

SYMPTOMS

- ☐ Distorted Vision
- ☐ Dizziness
- ☐ Irritability
- ☐ Light-headedness
- ☐ Light Sensitivity
- ☐ Malaise
- ☐ Nasal Congestion
- ☐ Nausea/Vomiting
- ☐ Sound Sensitivity
- ☐ Tender Scalp
- ☐
- ☐
- ☐

AURA (20-30 mins before)

- ☐ Black Spots
- ☐ Flashing Lights
- ☐ Lack of Vision
- ☐ Numbness FACE ARM LEG
- ☐ Zig Zag Lines
- ☐
- ☐

TRIGGER & SYMPTOM NOTES

REMEDIES

(NATURAL)

- ☐ Acupuncture
- ☐ Acupressure
- ☐ Caffeine
- ☐ Dark Room
- ☐ Hot Compress
- ☐ Hydration
- ☐
- ☐
- ☐
- ☐ Ice Pack
- ☐ Massage
- ☐ Relaxation
- ☐ Silence
- ☐ Walk
- ☐
- ☐
- ☐
- ☐

(OTC- COUNTER MEDS)

- ☐ Excedrin
- ☐ Ibuprofen
- ☐ Tylenol
- ☐
- ☐
- ☐
- ☐
- ☐
- ☐

(Rx - PREVENTIVE)

- ☐ Amitriptyline
- ☐ Atenolol
- ☐ Gabapentin
- ☐ Nurtriptyline
- ☐ Propranolol
- ☐ Topamax
- ☐ Valproate
- ☐
- ☐

(Rx - RELIEF)

- ☐ Naproxin
- ☐ Nurtec
- ☐ Sumatriptan
- ☐ Rizatriptan
- ☐ Ubrelvy
- ☐
- ☐

(SUPPLEMENTS)

- ☐ B2
- ☐ Butterbur
- ☐ Feverfew
- ☐ Magnesium
- ☐
- ☐
- ☐

WITHIN 1 HR OF PAIN YES NO PAIN RELIEF YES NO

REMEDY NOTES

IMPACT ON DAILY ACTIVITIES

NONE | MILD | MODERATE | SEVERE

WWW.ONEMINUTEMIGRAINEDIARY.COM

One Minute MIGRAINE Diary

Date : ______________

Start Time : ______________ End Time : ______________ Duration : ________

PAIN SCALE [1-10]	MENSTRUAL PERIOD	PAIN TYPE	WATER
1 2 3 4 5 6 7 8 9 10 MILD MODERATE SEVERE	YES NO Birth Control Pills YES NO	Stabbing Burning Pulsating Shocking Pressure Pounding SLEEP	MISSED MEALS YES NO
PAIN LOCATION FRONT BACK LEFT RIGHT TOP		WEATHER ° TEMP	STRESS YES NO
		LIGHTS YES NO SOUNDS YES NO	SMELLS YES NO

FOODS CONSUMED (within last 24 hours)	PRODROME (1-2 hours before headache)	SYMPTOMS	AURA (20-30 mins before)
☐ Alcohol	☐ Excessive Thirst	☐ Distorted Vision	☐ Black Spots
☐ Artificial Sweetener	☐ Excessive Yawning	☐ Dizziness	☐ Flashing Lights
☐ Beans	☐ Face Sensitivity	☐ Irritability	☐ Lack of Vision
☐ Caffeine	☐ Irritability	☐ Light-headedness	☐ Numbness FACE ARM LEG
☐ Cheese	☐ Light Sensitivity	☐ Light Sensitivity	☐ Zig Zag Lines
☐ Chocolate	☐ Neck Tightness	☐ Malaise	☐
☐ Fermented Foods	☐ Unexplained Fatigue	☐ Nasal Congestion	☐
☐ MSG	☐ Visual Disturbances	☐ Nausea/Vomiting	TRIGGER & SYMPTOM NOTES
☐ Non Friendly Fruits	☐	☐ Sound Sensitivity	
☐ Nuts	☐	☐ Tender Scalp	
☐ Processed Meats	☐	☐	
☐	☐	☐	
☐	☐	☐	
☐			

REMEDIES

(NATURAL)		(OTC- COUNTER MEDS)	(Rx - PREVENTIVE)	(Rx - RELIEF)	(SUPPLEMENTS)
☐ Acupuncture	☐ Ice Pack	☐ Excedrin	☐ Amitriptyline	☐ Naproxin	☐ B2
☐ Acupressure	☐ Massage	☐ Ibuprofen	☐ Atenolol	☐ Nurtec	☐ Butterbur
☐ Caffeine	☐ Relaxation	☐ Tylenol	☐ Gabapentin	☐ Sumatriptan	☐ Feverfew
☐ Dark Room	☐ Silence	☐	☐ Nurtriptyline	☐ Rizatriptan	☐ Magnesium
☐ Hot Compress	☐ Walk	☐	☐ Propranolol	☐ Ubrelvy	☐
☐ Hydration	☐	☐	☐ Topamax	☐	☐
☐	☐	☐	☐ Valproate	☐	☐
☐	☐	☐	☐	WITHIN 1 HR OF PAIN YES NO	PAIN RELIEF YES NO
☐	☐	☐	☐		

REMEDY NOTES

IMPACT ON DAILY ACTIVITIES

NONE | MILD | MODERATE | SEVERE

WWW.ONEMINUTEMIGRAINEDIARY.COM

One Minute MIGRAINE Diary

Date : ______________________

Start Time : ________________ End Time : ____________ Duration : ________

PAIN SCALE [1-10]

1 2 3 4 5 6 7 8 9 10

MILD MODERATE SEVERE

MENSTRUAL PERIOD

YES NO

Birth Control Pills

YES NO

PAIN TYPE

Stabbing Burning Pulsating Shocking Pressure Pounding

SLEEP

WATER

MISSED MEALS

YES NO

PAIN LOCATION

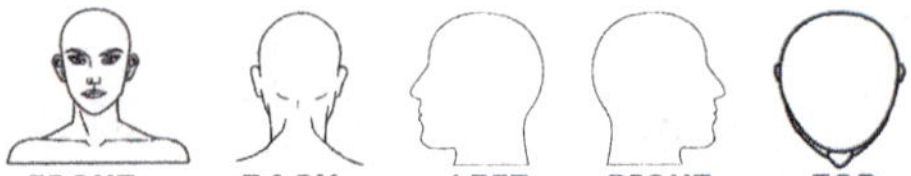

FRONT BACK LEFT RIGHT TOP

WEATHER

TEMP

STRESS

YES NO

LIGHTS

YES NO

SOUNDS

YES NO

SMELLS

YES NO

FOODS CONSUMED (within last 24 hours)

- ☐ Alcohol
- ☐ Artificial Sweetener
- ☐ Beans
- ☐ Caffeine
- ☐ Cheese
- ☐ Chocolate
- ☐ Fermented Foods
- ☐ MSG
- ☐ Non Friendly Fruits
- ☐ Nuts
- ☐ Processed Meats
- ☐
- ☐
- ☐

PRODROME (1-2 hours before headache)

- ☐ Excessive Thirst
- ☐ Excessive Yawning
- ☐ Face Sensitivity
- ☐ Irritability
- ☐ Light Sensitivity
- ☐ Neck Tightness
- ☐ Unexplained Fatigue
- ☐ Visual Disturbances
- ☐
- ☐
- ☐
- ☐
- ☐

SYMPTOMS

- ☐ Distorted Vision
- ☐ Dizziness
- ☐ Irritability
- ☐ Light-headedness
- ☐ Light Sensitivity
- ☐ Malaise
- ☐ Nasal Congestion
- ☐ Nausea/Vomiting
- ☐ Sound Sensitivity
- ☐ Tender Scalp
- ☐
- ☐
- ☐

AURA (20-30 mins before)

- ☐ Black Spots
- ☐ Flashing Lights
- ☐ Lack of Vision
- ☐ Numbness FACE ARM LEG
- ☐ Zig Zag Lines
- ☐
- ☐

TRIGGER & SYMPTOM NOTES

REMEDIES

(NATURAL)

- ☐ Acupuncture
- ☐ Acupressure
- ☐ Caffeine
- ☐ Dark Room
- ☐ Hot Compress
- ☐ Hydration
- ☐
- ☐
- ☐
- ☐ Ice Pack
- ☐ Massage
- ☐ Relaxation
- ☐ Silence
- ☐ Walk
- ☐
- ☐
- ☐
- ☐

(OTC- COUNTER MEDS)

- ☐ Excedrin
- ☐ Ibuprofen
- ☐ Tylenol
- ☐
- ☐
- ☐
- ☐
- ☐
- ☐

(Rx - PREVENTIVE)

- ☐ Amitriptyline
- ☐ Atenolol
- ☐ Gabapentin
- ☐ Nurtriptyline
- ☐ Propranolol
- ☐ Topamax
- ☐ Valproate
- ☐
- ☐

(Rx - RELIEF)

- ☐ Naproxin
- ☐ Nurtec
- ☐ Sumatriptan
- ☐ Rizatriptan
- ☐ Ubrelvy
- ☐
- ☐

(SUPPLEMENTS)

- ☐ B2
- ☐ Butterbur
- ☐ Feverfew
- ☐ Magnesium
- ☐
- ☐
- ☐

WITHIN 1 HR OF PAIN YES NO PAIN RELIEF YES NO

REMEDY NOTES

IMPACT ON DAILY ACTIVITIES

NONE | MILD | MODERATE | SEVERE

WWW.ONEMINUTEMIGRAINEDIARY.COM

One Minute MIGRAINE Diary

Date : ______________________

Start Time : ______________ End Time : ______________ Duration : ________

PAIN SCALE [1-10]	MENSTRUAL PERIOD	PAIN TYPE	WATER
1 2 3 4 5 6 7 8 9 10 MILD MODERATE SEVERE	YES NO Birth Control Pills YES NO	Stabbing Burning Pulsating Shocking Pressure Pounding **SLEEP**	**MISSED MEALS** YES NO

PAIN LOCATION

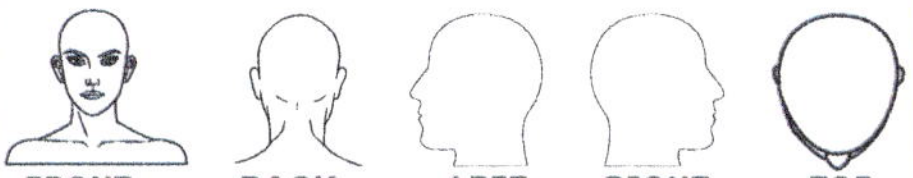

FRONT BACK LEFT RIGHT TOP

WEATHER

STRESS YES NO

LIGHTS YES NO

SOUNDS YES NO

SMELLS YES NO

FOODS CONSUMED (within last 24 hours)	PRODROME (1-2 hours before headache)	SYMPTOMS	AURA (20-30 mins before)
☐ Alcohol	☐ Excessive Thirst	☐ Distorted Vision	☐ Black Spots
☐ Artificial Sweetener	☐ Excessive Yawning	☐ Dizziness	☐ Flashing Lights
☐ Beans	☐ Face Sensitivity	☐ Irritability	☐ Lack of Vision
☐ Caffeine	☐ Irritability	☐ Light-headedness	☐ Numbness FACE ARM LEG
☐ Cheese	☐ Light Sensitivity	☐ Light Sensitivity	☐ Zig Zag Lines
☐ Chocolate	☐ Neck Tightness	☐ Malaise	☐
☐ Fermented Foods	☐ Unexplained Fatigue	☐ Nasal Congestion	☐
☐ MSG	☐ Visual Disturbances	☐ Nausea/Vomiting	**TRIGGER & SYMPTOM NOTES**
☐ Non Friendly Fruits	☐	☐ Sound Sensitivity	
☐ Nuts	☐	☐ Tender Scalp	
☐ Processed Meats	☐	☐	
☐	☐	☐	
☐	☐	☐	
☐	☐		

REMEDIES

(NATURAL)		(OTC- COUNTER MEDS)	(Rx - PREVENTIVE)	(Rx - RELIEF)	(SUPPLEMENTS)
☐ Acupuncture	☐ Ice Pack	☐ Excedrin	☐ Amitriptyline	☐ Naproxin	☐ B2
☐ Acupressure	☐ Massage	☐ Ibuprofen	☐ Atenolol	☐ Nurtec	☐ Butterbur
☐ Caffeine	☐ Relaxation	☐ Tylenol	☐ Gabapentin	☐ Sumatriptan	☐ Feverfew
☐ Dark Room	☐ Silence	☐	☐ Nurtriptyline	☐ Rizatriptan	☐ Magnesium
☐ Hot Compress	☐ Walk	☐	☐ Propranolol	☐ Ubrelvy	☐
☐ Hydration	☐	☐	☐ Topamax	☐	☐
☐	☐	☐	☐ Valproate	☐	☐
☐	☐	☐	☐	WITHIN 1 HR OF PAIN YES NO	PAIN RELIEF YES NO
☐	☐	☐	☐		

REMEDY NOTES

IMPACT ON DAILY ACTIVITIES

NONE | MILD | MODERATE | SEVERE

WWW.ONEMINUTEMIGRAINEDIARY.COM

One Minute MIGRAINE Diary

Date : ____________________

Start Time : ______________ End Time : ______________ Duration : __________

PAIN SCALE [1-10]

|-----|-----|-----|-----|-----|-----|-----|-----|-----|
1 2 3 4 5 6 7 8 9 10
MILD MODERATE SEVERE

MENSTRUAL PERIOD
YES NO
Birth Control Pills
YES NO

PAIN TYPE
Stabbing Burning Pulsating Shocking Pressure Pounding

SLEEP

WATER

MISSED MEALS
YES NO

PAIN LOCATION

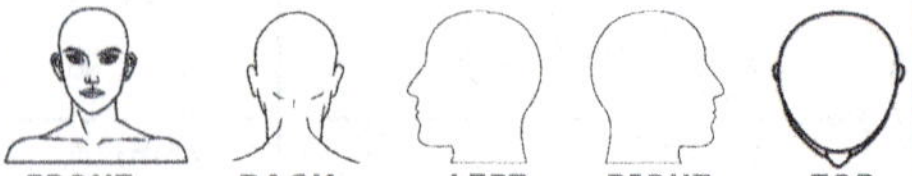

FRONT BACK LEFT RIGHT TOP

WEATHER
° TEMP

STRESS
YES NO

LIGHTS
YES NO

SOUNDS
YES NO

SMELLS
YES NO

FOODS CONSUMED
(within last 24 hours)

- ☐ Alcohol
- ☐ Artificial Sweetener
- ☐ Beans
- ☐ Caffeine
- ☐ Cheese
- ☐ Chocolate
- ☐ Fermented Foods
- ☐ MSG
- ☐ Non Friendly Fruits
- ☐ Nuts
- ☐ Processed Meats
- ☐
- ☐
- ☐

PRODROME
(1-2 hours before headache)

- ☐ Excessive Thirst
- ☐ Excessive Yawning
- ☐ Face Sensitivity
- ☐ Irritability
- ☐ Light Sensitivity
- ☐ Neck Tightness
- ☐ Unexplained Fatigue
- ☐ Visual Disturbances
- ☐
- ☐
- ☐
- ☐
- ☐

SYMPTOMS

- ☐ Distorted Vision
- ☐ Dizziness
- ☐ Irritability
- ☐ Light-headedness
- ☐ Light Sensitivity
- ☐ Malaise
- ☐ Nasal Congestion
- ☐ Nausea/Vomiting
- ☐ Sound Sensitivity
- ☐ Tender Scalp
- ☐
- ☐
- ☐

AURA
(20-30 mins before)

- ☐ Black Spots
- ☐ Flashing Lights
- ☐ Lack of Vision
- ☐ Numbness FACE ARM LEG
- ☐ Zig Zag Lines
- ☐
- ☐

TRIGGER & SYMPTOM NOTES

REMEDIES

(NATURAL)

- ☐ Acupuncture
- ☐ Acupressure
- ☐ Caffeine
- ☐ Dark Room
- ☐ Hot Compress
- ☐ Hydration
- ☐
- ☐
- ☐
- ☐ Ice Pack
- ☐ Massage
- ☐ Relaxation
- ☐ Silence
- ☐ Walk
- ☐
- ☐
- ☐
- ☐

(OTC- COUNTER MEDS)

- ☐ Excedrin
- ☐ Ibuprofen
- ☐ Tylenol
- ☐
- ☐
- ☐
- ☐
- ☐
- ☐

(Rx - PREVENTIVE)

- ☐ Amitriptyline
- ☐ Atenolol
- ☐ Gabapentin
- ☐ Nurtriptyline
- ☐ Propranolol
- ☐ Topamax
- ☐ Valproate
- ☐
- ☐

(Rx - RELIEF)

- ☐ Naproxin
- ☐ Nurtec
- ☐ Sumatriptan
- ☐ Rizatriptan
- ☐ Ubrelvy
- ☐
- ☐

(SUPPLEMENTS)

- ☐ B2
- ☐ Butterbur
- ☐ Feverfew
- ☐ Magnesium
- ☐
- ☐
- ☐

WITHIN 1 HR OF PAIN YES NO PAIN RELIEF YES NO

REMEDY NOTES

IMPACT ON DAILY ACTIVITIES
NONE | MILD | MODERATE | SEVERE

WWW.ONEMINUTEMIGRAINEDIARY.COM

One Minute MIGRAINE Diary

Date : ______________________

Start Time : ______________ End Time : ____________ Duration : ________

PAIN SCALE [1-10]	MENSTRUAL PERIOD	PAIN TYPE	WATER
1 2 3 4 5 6 7 8 9 10 MILD MODERATE SEVERE	YES NO Birth Control Pills YES NO	Stabbing Burning Pulsating Shocking Pressure Pounding SLEEP	MISSED MEALS YES NO
PAIN LOCATION FRONT BACK LEFT RIGHT TOP		WEATHER ° TEMP	STRESS YES NO
		LIGHTS YES NO SOUNDS YES NO	SMELLS YES NO

FOODS CONSUMED (within last 24 hours)	PRODROME (1-2 hours before headache)	SYMPTOMS	AURA (20-30 mins before)
☐ Alcohol	☐ Excessive Thirst	☐ Distorted Vision	☐ Black Spots
☐ Artificial Sweetener	☐ Excessive Yawning	☐ Dizziness	☐ Flashing Lights
☐ Beans	☐ Face Sensitivity	☐ Irritability	☐ Lack of Vision
☐ Caffeine	☐ Irritability	☐ Light-headedness	☐ Numbness FACE ARM LEG
☐ Cheese	☐ Light Sensitivity	☐ Light Sensitivity	☐ Zig Zag Lines
☐ Chocolate	☐ Neck Tightness	☐ Malaise	☐
☐ Fermented Foods	☐ Unexplained Fatigue	☐ Nasal Congestion	☐
☐ MSG	☐ Visual Disturbances	☐ Nausea/Vomiting	TRIGGER & SYMPTOM NOTES
☐ Non Friendly Fruits	☐	☐ Sound Sensitivity	
☐ Nuts	☐	☐ Tender Scalp	
☐ Processed Meats	☐	☐	
☐	☐	☐	
☐	☐	☐	
☐			

REMEDIES

(NATURAL)		(OTC- COUNTER MEDS)	(Rx - PREVENTIVE)	(Rx - RELIEF)	(SUPPLEMENTS)
☐ Acupuncture	☐ Ice Pack	☐ Excedrin	☐ Amitriptyline	☐ Naproxin	☐ B2
☐ Acupressure	☐ Massage	☐ Ibuprofen	☐ Atenolol	☐ Nurtec	☐ Butterbur
☐ Caffeine	☐ Relaxation	☐ Tylenol	☐ Gabapentin	☐ Sumatriptan	☐ Feverfew
☐ Dark Room	☐ Silence	☐	☐ Nurtriptyline	☐ Rizatriptan	☐ Magnesium
☐ Hot Compress	☐ Walk	☐	☐ Propranolol	☐ Ubrelvy	☐
☐ Hydration	☐	☐	☐ Topamax	☐	☐
☐	☐	☐	☐ Valproate	☐	☐
☐	☐	☐	☐	WITHIN 1 HR OF PAIN YES NO	PAIN RELIEF YES NO
☐	☐	☐	☐		

REMEDY NOTES

IMPACT ON DAILY ACTIVITIES

NONE | MILD | MODERATE | SEVERE

WWW.ONEMINUTEMIGRAINEDIARY.COM

One Minute MIGRAINE Diary

MONTHLY REPORT

Monthly and Annual Migraine Tracking Reflections and Reviews Help You Track and Manage Your Migraines

WWW.ONEMINUTEMIGRAINEDIARY.COM

I am not my pain
My pain does not define me
I am not my pain
I am not defined by my pain
I am not my pain
I am strong, capable and confident

Book MEDIA Services

MONTHLY MIGRAINE *Report*

Month/ Year : ________________

KEY : M (Mild) MO(Moderate) S(Severe)

		KEY	TOP DAILY TRIGGERS
	1		
TOP MONTHLY TRIGGERS	2		
	3		
	4		
	5		
	6		
	7		
	8		
	9		
	10		
	11		
	12		
	13		
	14		
	15		
	16		
	17		
	18		
	19		
	20		
	21		
	22		
	23		
	24		
	25		
	26		
	27		
	28		
	29		
	30		
	31		

MONTHLY TOTAL:

WWW.ONEMINUTEMIGRAINEDIARY.COM

MONTHLY MIGRAINE Report

Month/ Year : ____________ KEY : M (Mild) MO(Moderate) S(Severe)

		KEY	TOP DAILY TRIGGERS
	1		
TOP MONTHLY TRIGGERS	2		
	3		
	4		
	5		
	6		
	7		
	8		
	9		
	10		
	11		
	12		
	13		
	14		
	15		
	16		
	17		
	18		
	19		
	20		
	21		
	22		
	23		
	24		
	25		
	26		
	27		
	28		
	29		
	30		
	31		

MONTHLY TOTAL:

WWW.ONEMINUTEMIGRAINEDIARY.COM

MONTHLY MIGRAINE Report

Month/ Year : ______________

KEY : M (Mild) MO(Moderate) S(Severe)

		KEY	TOP DAILY TRIGGERS
	1		
TOP MONTHLY TRIGGERS	2		
	3		
	4		
	5		
	6		
	7		
	8		
	9		
	10		
	11		
	12		
	13		
	14		
	15		
	16		
	17		
	18		
	19		
	20		
	21		
	22		
	23		
	24		
	25		
	26		
	27		
	28		
	29		
	30		
	31		

MONTHLY TOTAL:

WWW.ONEMINUTEMIGRAINEDIARY.COM

One Minute MIGRAINE Diary

ANNUAL REPORT

Monthly and Annual Migraine Tracking Reflections and Reviews Help You Track and Manage Your Migraines

WWW.ONEMINUTEMIGRAINEDIARY.COM

ANNUAL MIGRAINE Report

Year : ____________

KEY : M (Mild) MO(Moderate) S(Severe)

TOP MONTHLY TRIGGERS		J	F	M	A	M	J	J	A	S	O	N	D
	1												
	2												
	3												
	4												
	5												
	6												
	7												
	8												
	9												
	10												
	11												
	12												
TOP ANNUAL TRIGGERS	13												
	14												
	15												
	16												
	17												
	18												
	19												
	20												
	21												
	22												
	23												
	24												
	25												
	26												
	27												
	28												
	29												
	30												
	31												
TOTAL / MONTH													

GRAND TOTAL:

WWW.ONEMINUTEMIGRAINEDIARY.COM

ANNUAL MIGRAINE Report

Year : ____________

KEY : M (Mild) MO(Moderate) S(Severe)

TOP MONTHLY TRIGGERS		J	F	M	A	M	J	J	A	S	O	N	D
	1												
	2												
	3												
	4												
	5												
	6												
	7												
	8												
	9												
	10												
	11												
	12												
TOP ANNUAL TRIGGERS	13												
	14												
	15												
	16												
	17												
	18												
	19												
	20												
	21												
	22												
	23												
	24												
	25												
	26												
	27												
	28												
	29												
	30												
	31												
TOTAL / MONTH													

GRAND TOTAL:

WWW.ONEMINUTEMIGRAINEDIARY.COM

One Minute MIGRAINE Diary

Your Discovery

Review Reports, Analyze and Act

Analyze

If you committed to recording your migraines on a daily basis for 90 days, we are certain that you were able to discover a few lifestyle, environmental, or food triggers that bring on or worsen your migriaines.

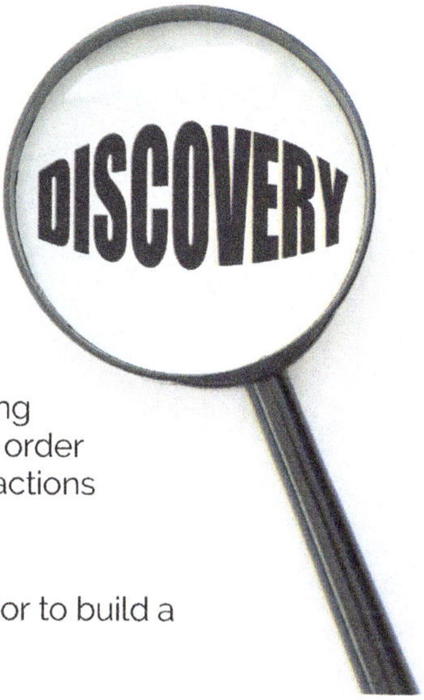

Act

Once you make new discoveries regarding your migraines, it is time to take action in order to manage them better. Here are some actions you can take.

- ✓ Discuss your finding with your doctor to build a headache management plan
- ✓ Try to eliminate or minimize triggers that cause headaches. These may include lifestyle changes, stress management, environmental and diet changes
- ✓ Adjust therapeutic, preventative, and acute remedies to find the one that works best for you

One Minute MIGRAINE Diary

Thank You...

Thank you for using the one-minute migraine diary to log your migraines. Our goal is to make tracking migraines easy and efficient. We would love to hear from you if you have any ideas to make this product even better for the migraine warriors around the world.

You can reach us at
hello@oneminutemigrainediary.com

Warmly,
One Minute Migraine Diary Team

WWW.ONEMINUTEMIGRAINEDIARY.COM

Made in the USA
Monee, IL
03 November 2026

67375725R00079